I0790860

WELCOME

So glad you decided to do something to help kids eat healthy and be more active in your community. With the help of this guidebook you can play the pivotal role in getting Kiwanis Righturn.Club at your local school or other organization.

This mentor led fitness program begins with you. Read through this guidebook, apply the information supplied here and you are on your way to making your own right turn.

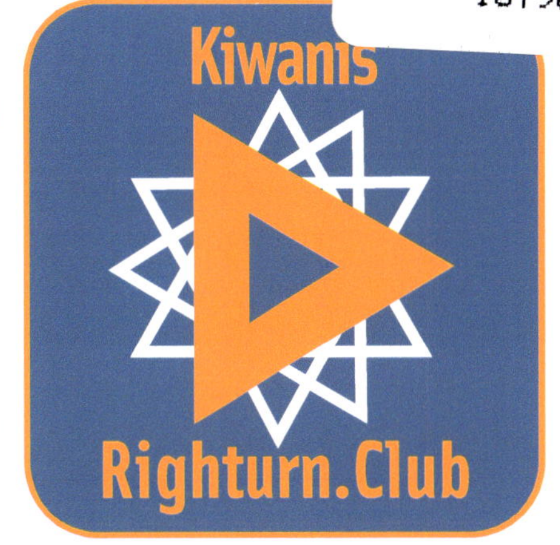

The inaugural program began in the spring of 2016 at Sutter Creek Elementary School in Sutter Creek, California. The 10 week program met after school twice a week for two hours. 28 Local volunteers helped make this happen including high school students, local Kiwanis Club members, parents and others from the community. We repeat the program every spring and fall, now starting our 5th season, fall 2017. The results will be the lasting effect Kiwanis Righturn.Club will have on all the participants, from the kids and their families to the volunteers and Kiwanians.

ABOUT THE AUTHOR

Thomas Moraitis is the Founder of Kiwanis Righturn.Club and resides in Sutter Creek, California near Sacramento in the foothills of the Sierra's. He is the father of Timothy and Terah who witnessed Thomas transform from 234 lbs to 164 lbs. He has kept the weight off for over 10 years using the principles outlined in this Guidebook.

He received a BA and MA at California Start University, Fullerton. His career began as a teacher in Anaheim,California. His work continued with children after teaching, with the design of Jacques Cousteau's *Dolphin Log*, a magazine for elementary age kids. Previously to working full

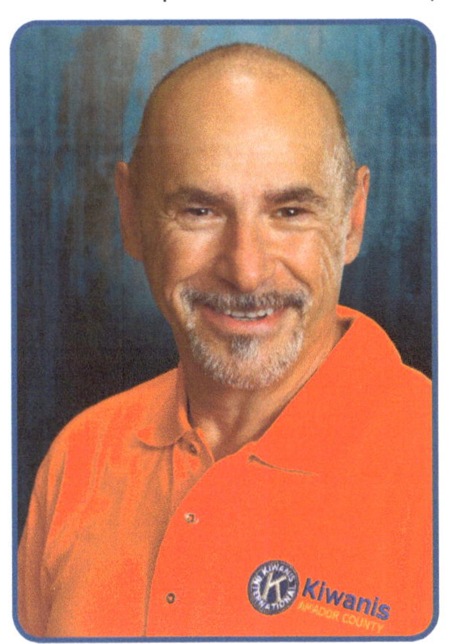

time on Righturn.Club he led his own Design Firm, TM Design Group in Orange County, California. He then served as Creative Director at Citrix Online, Apartments.com and MyPoints.com.

He was a member of Kiwanis Key Club at Highland Park High School in Detroit, Michigan in 1967 and Savanna High School, in Anaheim, California to 1969. Fifty years later he uncovered a 50 year Kiwanis Medal and noticed it has now been 100 years. He joined Kiwanis Amador County in 2015 and now serves as 2017 President.

Contact Info: Thomas@Righturn.Club

PO Box 1853, Sutter Creek, CA 95685

"There is nothing wrong with change, if it is in the right direction." Winston Churchill

Text Copyright ©2017 by Thomas Moraitis. Photo's used by permission.
ISBN: 13 978-1542599757

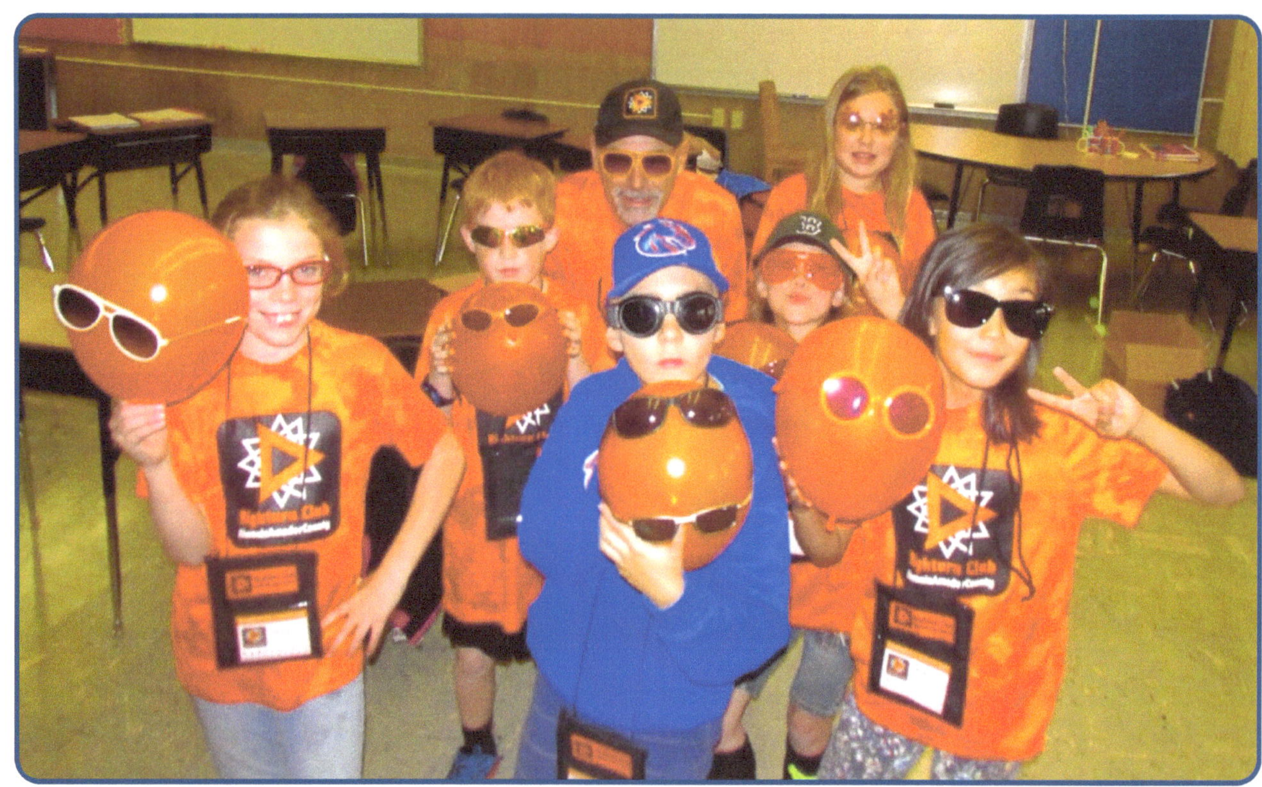

Sunglass Day at Sutter Creek Elementary School Kiwanis Righturn.Club

CREATIVE RESOURCES

CONTENTS

STARTING A CLUB?

Please let Thomas Moraitis know if you start a club.

Email: Thomas@Righturn.Club

Mail: Thomas Moraitis, PO Box 1853, Sutter Creek, CA 95685

Comments,questions and photos are welcome. Like us on FaceBook: Righturn.Club

Giving Thanks

Heartfelt thanks goes to all those involved in creating Kiwanis Righturn.Club: members, mentors, volunteers, friends, Kiwanis Club members near and far.

▶ **Anne Illgen,** who was my first mentor, who walked, ran, swam and biked with me, in 2006. A coworker at Citrix Online. She helped me lose 70 lbs. From 234 to 164, going on 10 years.

▶ **Joe Cato,** Race Director for the Santa Barbara Triathlon who encouraged me on my journey to health and fitness, during those transforming years.

▶ **Kevin Blasingame,** Kiwanis Amador County Member for supporting my passion to help kids and providing funding for the program.

▶ **Roberta Ross,** Kiwanis Amador County Member, Volunteer Mentor, who has brought her expertise and knowledge to help kids understand health and fitness, and for editing Kiwanis Righturn.Club Training Manual.

▶ **Sean Snider,** School Principal of Sutter Creek Elementary for hosting our first club, encouraging students to participate and for welcoming us back each year.

▶ **Christina Hermanson,** Parent and Volunteer for helping the entire 10 weeks at Sutter Creek Elementary School and giving her insight into bringing order and consistency in working with kids.

▶ **Guy Blair,** Kiwanis Amador County Member who traveled from Carmichael, CA. to Sutter Creek beginning in Fall, 2016 to assist as a mentor leader. He is my mentor when it comes to leadership and Kiwanis relations.

▶ **Jeffrey Lapid,** for filming the first Kiwanis Righturn.Club activities in Sutter Creek, CA.

▶ **David Ingram,** for his support and adding his chef experience to our healthy snack and drink menu.

▶ **Theressa Moraitis, Timothy Moraitis and Terah Moraitis Hagy,** who helped create this program and were my constant source of encouragement in improving my health and fitness.

▶ **All the kids,** for their joy motivation and participation.

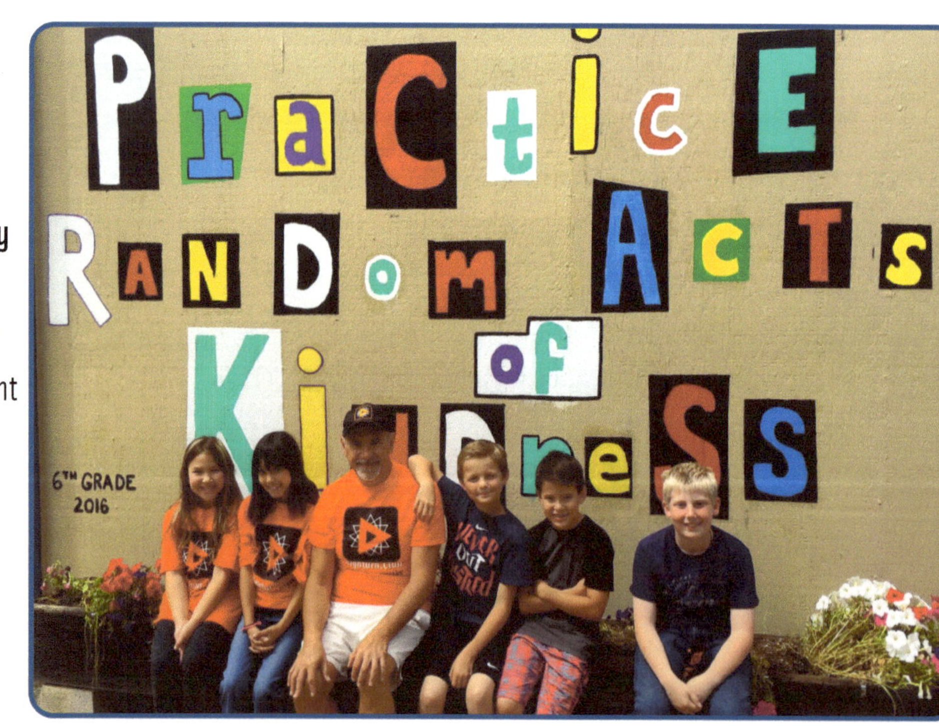

The Right Need

What can we do to help kids age 8-12 today that will have the greatest impact for their future well being? What can help them make healthier choices when it comes to health and fitness? Kiwanis Righturn.Club does just that. Did you know that...*

▶ ...38% of 5th graders in California are overweight or obese?

▶ ...75% of overweight teens are likely to be obese as adults.

▶ ...80% of children diagnosed with type 2 diabetes are overweight.

▶ ...California ranks #1 among all states in the amount it spends on the health consequences of obesity.

▶ ...Obesity rates have increased considerably in the last 30 years: 4 times higher among 6-11 year olds. *Source: www.publichealthadvocacy.org

The Right Time

Elementary age kids are the perfect age to start lifelong practices that will last a lifetime. They learn to read, to write, to play, to share and to be kind. They can also learn to excel in physical activities and to know what's best when it comes to eating right. They can also influence their families, friends and neighbors and all they come into contact with and become mentors. Kiwanis Righturn.Club is a training ground for future leaders and mentors.

The Right Value

What matters most is the opportunity to bring to these kids the tools that will enable them to excel still more regardless of their endeavors. The true value of Kiwanis Righturn.Club is that when you mix 3 things: fun, simple truths and actions —it works. *It is not an exercise program or a diet. It's a lifestyle.*

In 2009, I founded a similar program, ZultzClub, Mentor Led Fitness in Ventura, California. Zultz was short for results. We met at Sheridan Way Elementary School and 3 years after the 10 week program was completed I ran into one of the kids, Luis at a grocery store on Ventura Ave. He was with his mother, who spoke no English. Luis said, "Hi Mr. M., I'm on the football team." I recognized his face and remembered how big he WAS. He looked like a normal Middle School student now. His mother said, "ZultzClub, ZultzClub!" and motioned with her hands up and down her sons body with the palm of her hands parallel, indicating how skinny her son is.

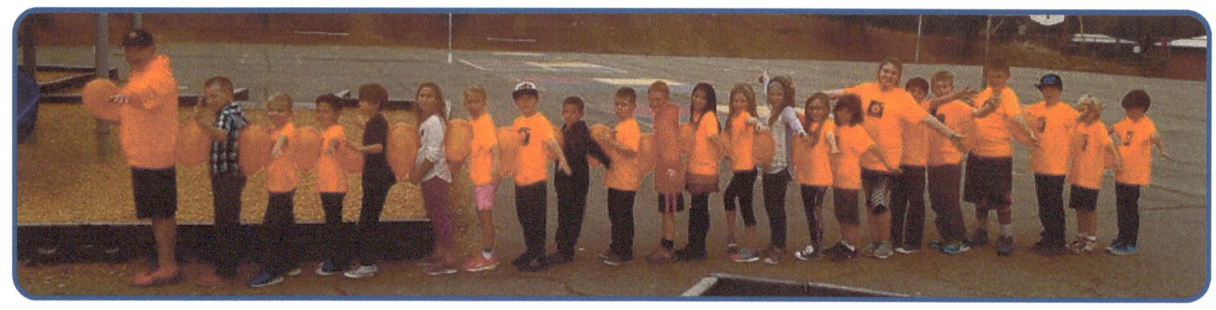

Kiwanis Righturn.Club Fall 2017 at Sutter Creek Elementary School: Orange Balloon Caterpillar Game

It took 7 years to bring the program back. The name was changed from ZultzClub to Righturn.Club. It was after joining Kiwanis Amador County and being asked, "What is your passion for children?" I said, "I want to focus on helping kids who are obese, and can't help themselves. It's not their fault. They can make a simple right turn, and change the direction of their lives. Will you help me to reach out to these kids?" The Kiwanians asked for a proposal, and agreed to fund the first program in Sutter Creek, California. For 10 weeks, we met at Sutter Creek Elementary School and reached kids and their families with this program. Parents, teachers, volunteers from the community, Kiwanians and high school kids, 28 people total, helped bring this to fruition. We met in the spring of 2016 after spring break to the end of the school year. Jeffrey Lapid, a Sacramento area videographer filmed the kids running, eating healthy snacks, preparing food, drinks, playing games, dancing, having fun and talking. The Kiwanis Righturn.Club Documentary Film, is available for showing. Contact Thomas Moraitis.

It is now the Fall of 2017, and the new principle, James Hamilton is welcoming us back. We are including 3rd thru 6th graders.

Delegate, delegate, delegate! You, as the chief organizer cannot do everything. So in looking at your volunteers, see what areas they would like to help in. Visit the local high school to recruit some runners to keep up with the fast kids. Use the sign up sheet for key volunteers for each meeting. Volunteers can sign up for one or more meetings. Local Kiwanians can also sign up. Bring the sign up sheet to one of their meetings. Look at your social areas, and, most of all, have fun.

The Right Image

All the items included in the manual were designed by Thomas Moraitis. After a career of designing for organizations and companies, Thomas brought his design abilities to this program. The logo has several layers of meaning. The orange triangle points to the right and has three corners. It is also the symbol of power on. The white triangles show movement, and change of direction, the aim of Kiwanis Righturn.Club. The name is also the website URL. Combining two triangles form the Star of David, representing his faith. Orange is his favorite color and symbolizes health, vitality and positive energy. It is also the color for safety and when the kids run on the streets they are very visible. Kiwanis Righturn.Club is the signature project of Kiwanis Amador County.

CHAPTER 1

Starting a Righturn.Club

It's easier than you think. Here are the 12 steps.

►   1. Read this training manual and learn what Kiwanis Righturn.Club is.

►   2. Identify a local elementary school in your area.

►   3. Meet with the Principal and ask if a Kiwanis Righturn.Club would meet the need for an after shool program. Is there a room available for use after shool?

►   4. Determine a 10 week time period with the Principal. Decide on days.

►   5. Contact a Kiwanis Club in the same area. Meet with the President.

►   6. Submit a proposal to the local Kiwanis Club for a $1,000. budget approval.

►   7. Once approved, recruit volunteers to help. Have mentors complete application.

►   8. Give the school a *Student Application Form* to reproduce and send home.

►   9. Meet with each potential class, handout flyer to get the buzz going.

►   10. Make arrangements at your local food bank for weekly snack pick up.

►   11. Follow school district and Kiwanis guidelines for volunteers to ensure children's security.

►   12. Order shirts, print name tags, buy games as noted. Schedule helpers.

There you go. Easy does it. The handout for classroom visits it on the next page, titled, ALL RIGHT.

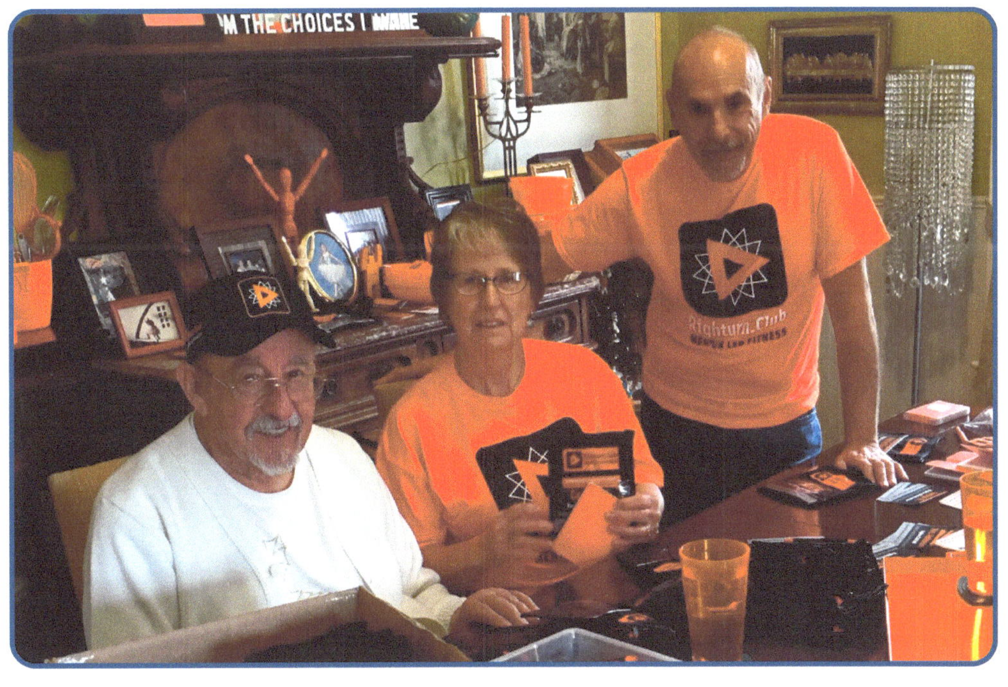

Volunteers Melody and Dick Anderson from Kiwanis of Amador County preparing for Kiwanis Righturn.Club at Sutter Creek Elementary School

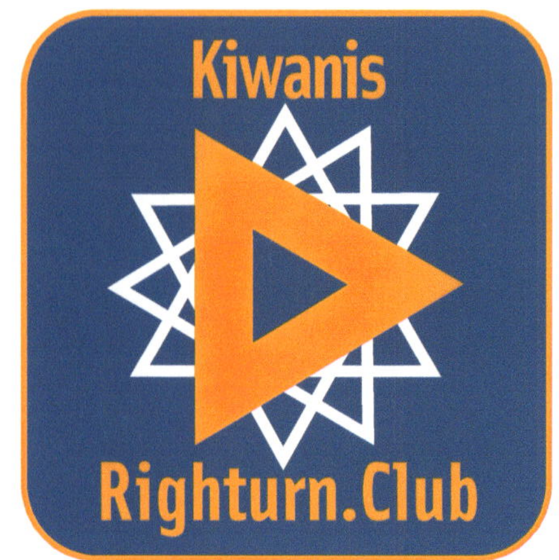

ALL RIGHT!

School:______________________

Time:______________________

Dates:______________________

Become a Member of Righturn.Club

Run, play games, eat and hang out with friends!

I'm ______________________________________ **I'm in** __________ **Grade**

I love to eat and drink...

Use words or drawings of your favorites inside shirt.

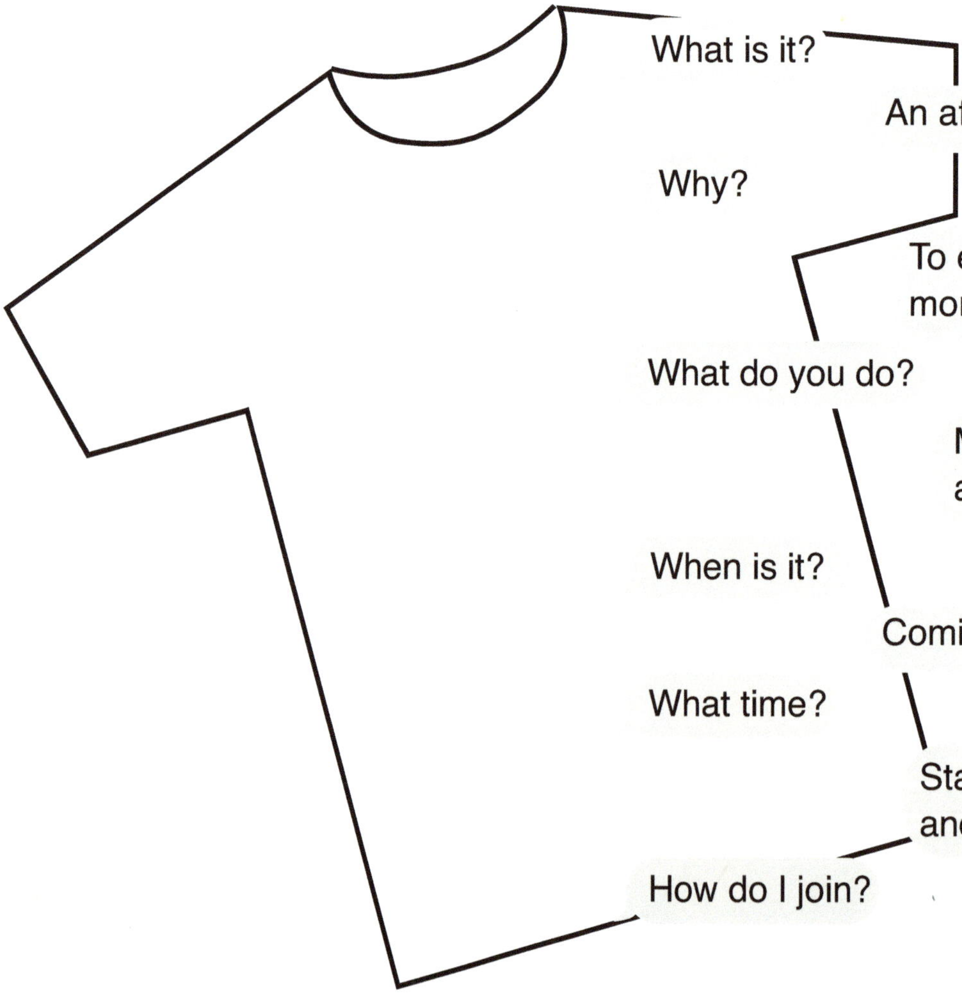

What is it?

An afterschool running club.

Why?

To eat healthier and be more active and have fun!

What do you do?

Meet, dance, play, run and get free snacks.

When is it?

Coming soon at this school.

What time?

Starts right after school and goes for 2 hours.

How do I join?

Sign up, get your parents permission

Contact Info:______________________________

CHAPTER 2

Righturn.Club Volunteer Sign Up Sheet

VOLUNTEER!

School:_________________

Time:_________________

Dates:_________________

▶ Days: Mon/Wed or Tues/Thurs (Circle One)

▶ Dates from ______________ to ______________

▶ Volunteer for one or more days. Thank You!

Job A: Volunteer. Responsibilities include overseeing children's snack preparation, assisting in activities, encouraging the kids: 2 Hours

Job B: Mentor Volunteer. Responsibilities include meeting with kids, leading a chat on a healthy topic (content provided) and running/ walking: 2 Hours

Job A or B	Dates	Name	Email	Phone
1. _____	1. ______________	________________	________________	___________
2. _____	2. ______________	________________	________________	___________
3. _____	3. ______________	________________	________________	___________
4. _____	4. ______________	________________	________________	___________
5. _____	5. ______________	________________	________________	___________
6. _____	6. ______________	________________	________________	___________
7. _____	7. ______________	________________	________________	___________
8. _____	8. ______________	________________	________________	___________
9. _____	9. ______________	________________	________________	___________
10. ____	10. _____________	________________	________________	___________
11. ____	11. _____________	________________	________________	___________
12. ____	12. _____________	________________	________________	___________
13. ____	13. _____________	________________	________________	___________
14. ____	14. _____________	________________	________________	___________
15. ____	15. _____________	________________	________________	___________
16. ____	16. _____________	________________	________________	___________
17. ____	17. _____________	________________	________________	___________
18. ____	18. _____________	________________	________________	___________
19. ____	19. _____________	________________	________________	___________
20. ____	20. _____________	________________	________________	___________

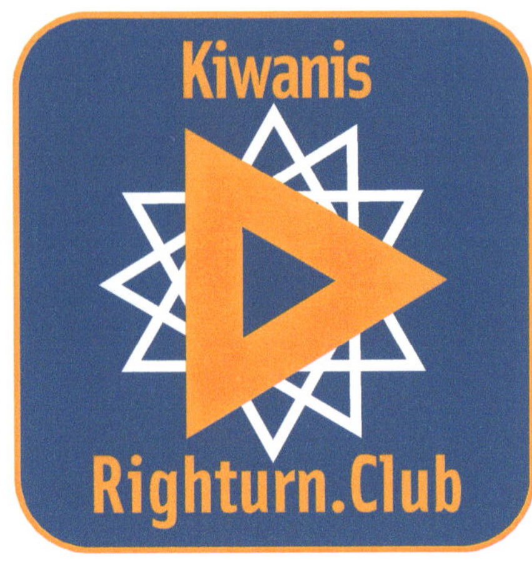

VOLUNTEER!

School:_________________

Time:_________________

Dates:_________________

Help Kids Get Fit and Choose Healthy

Call for Mentors and Community Volunteers

The Need To Make A Right Turn

▶ Are you ready to give back to your community? Do you have some free time for the 10 weeks mentioned above?

▶ We are the choices we make. Help kids be more active and make better choices with your help as a mentor.

▶ It's time to do what's right! Right now!

Righturn.Club Is...

▶ ...a fitness program focused on kids who want to get fit and make better food choices with the help of a Mentor.

▶ ...kids meet with Mentors (teens and adults from the community) after school, twice a week for 10 weeks.

▶ ...where you will give a short chat on health and fitness.

▶ ...a way for kids to get fit and learn about healthy eating.

▶ ...also a place where others, besides mentors, can join in and help, take roll, and assist where needed.

What Happens at a Righturn.Club Meeting?

▶ ON YOUR MARK: Children check in and meet their Mentor.

▶ GET SET: Each lesson has a theme. The Mentor asks a question and then shares a few facts.

▶ Righturn.Club AEROBICS: Everyone warms up, and moves! A dance is learned or a game is played.

▶ Kids and Mentors run together on a preset set course. They run, they walk, everyone gets stronger and faster while having fun and being a part of the club.

▶ Kids and Mentors eat a healthy snack and drink together.

How to Volunteer in Righturn.Club

▶ Fill out the Mentor Application Form

▶ Don't delay. You may be required to do a fingerprint scan, a TB test and Mentor Training before meeting the kids.

▶ All volunteers are welcome, regardless of age, size, shape or degree of fitness.

▶ Volunteer TODAY for 2 to 20 meetings! Any help is appreciated.

CHAPTER 3

Applications for Members, Mentors and Volunteers

Sample applications follow, they may be personalized for the local school and Kiwanis Club Sponsor. The questions asked will help in administrating the program. As the leader, you need to be aware of any special needs, know who to call in case of an emergency and be cleared of any liability for all involved. If you want to take pictures, you need a signed parent permission. Never use the childs last name in promotional materials.

Some ideas for recruitment of volunteers include local health clubs, health fairs or any place where fitness is encouraged. You can also attend a Parent Teacher Meeting with permission from the principle to recruit parent volunteers. Often times, parents pick up their children, and you can say hello, and ask if they can come early a time or two to help.

Teachers make excellent volunteers, as they are already at the location. They often know the kids by name, and if they are into health, fitness, love to run it's a natural fit.

Once the student applications are received, the school should keep one copy and give a copy to you. This is kept in a binder, in the designated meeting area, for emergency use. The information is confidential and should be treated with respect. You could also create an email list, being sure to always use blind CC, so email addresses are not shared if communications to parents is needed. I prefer sending a flyer or "invite" home with the students.

I found by asking only for sign ups for a specific meeting, not ALL is easier for recruiting. I also found that once a parent or volunteers, they want to come again. We had Tuesday volunteers, Thursday volunteers, and occasional or fill-in volunteers,for those that had other things going. We never lacked help, even in our small town.

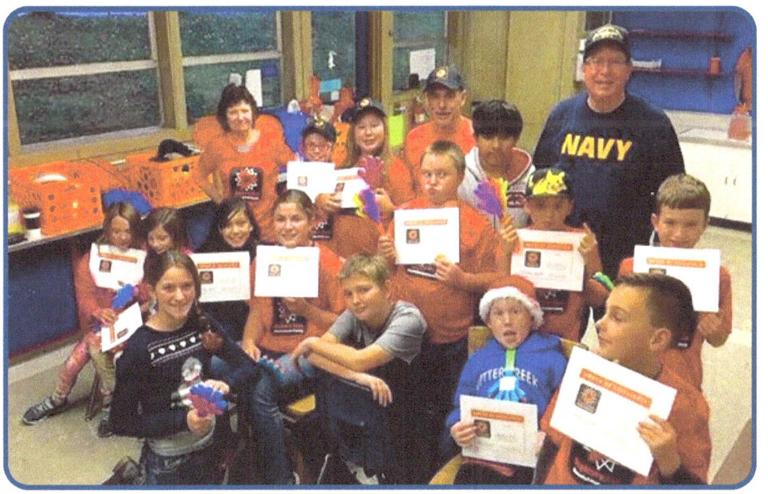

Roberta Ross, Thomas Moraitis, and Guy Blair at the Award
Presentations at Sutter Creek Elementary School, Fall 2016.

"The time is always RIGHT to do what is RIGHT."

Martin Luther King, Jr.

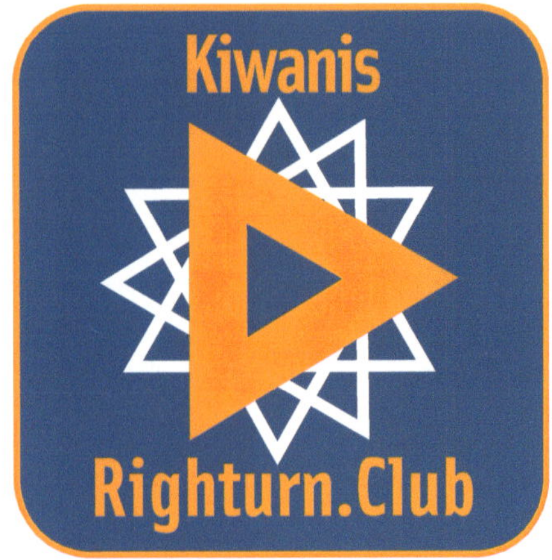

APPLICATION

School:_____________________

Time:_____________________

Dates:_____________________

Righturn.Club Student Information
Información del Alumno

▶ **Last Name** Apellido_____________________ **First Name** Nombre_____________________

Middle Name Apellido_____________________ **Date of Birth** Fecha de Nacimiento_____________________

Name of School Nombre de la Escuela Sutter Creek Elementary School

Home Street Address Dirección_____________________**City, State, Zip** Ciudad, Estado, Zona Postal_____________________

Home Telephone Teléfono de la Casa_____________________**Cell Phone** Celular_____________________

What language do adults most frequently use at home? Que idioma usan los adultos más frecuentemente en el hogar?_____________________

▶ **Legal Father** Informacion del Padre O Tutor: **Name** Nombre_____________________

Address, if different from above Dirección si es diferente que la anterior **Home Street Address** Dirección_____________________

City, State, Zip Ciudad, Estado, Zona Postal_____________________

Home Street Address Dirección_____________________**City, State, Zip** Ciudad, Estado, Zona Postal_____________________

Employer Name Empleado del Padre_____________________**Work Phone Number** Teléfono del trabajo_____________________

Email Dirección de Correo Electrónico_____________________

▶ **Legal Mother** Información de la Madre o Tutora: **Name** Nombre_____________________

Address, if different from above Dirección si es diferente de la anterior **Home Street Address** Dirección_____________________

City, State, Zip Ciudad, Estado, Zona Postal_____________________

Home Street Address Dirección_____________________**City, State, Zip** Ciudad, Estado, Zona Postal_____________________

Employer Name Empleador de la Madre_____________________**Work Phone Number** Teléfono del trabajo_____________________

Email Dirección del correo Electronico_____________________

▶ **Additional Emergency Contact** Para Contactoen Caso de Emergencia: **In the event of illness, medical emergency, disaster or the Parent/Legal Guardian cannot be reached, a school official may call the following friends, relatives or adult siblings 18 and over, who are authorized to take responsisility for the student's care:** En caso de enfermedad, emergencia médica o desastre, y, si no se puede localizar a los padres o tutores, un funcionario de la escuela podrá llamar a los siguientes amigos o parientes adultos, de 18 anos o mayores, los cuales están autorizados a tomar responsabilidad el cuidado del estudiante:

▶ **Name of Childcare Provider** Nombre de la persona encargada del cuidado del nino(a)_____________________

Name Nombre_____________________**Address** Dirección_____________________**Phone** Teléfono_____________________

Relationship Parentesco_____________________**Home Telephone** Teléfono de Casa_____________________**Cell** Celular_____________________

Please Complete Other Side. Complete por favor el otro lado también.

▶ **Health Information** Información del Padre O Tutor: **Please complete the health information below. Check all that apply.** Favor de completer la historia clinica que se le solicita: marque donde corresponda:

___ **Allergies, Include Type, food, bee, etc.** Alergia, indique de qué tipo: alimentos, abejas, etc:_______________________

___ **Asthma** Asma **Describe**_________________________________Describa_______________________

___ **Diabetes** Diabetes **Describe**_________________________________Describa_______________________

___ **Heart Problem** Problemas del corazon **Describe**_______________________Describa_______________________

___ **Hemophilia** Hemofilia **Describe**_________________________Describa_______________________

___ **Other Health Concerns or Special Needs** Otros problemas de salud_______________________________________

▶ **Parent/Guardian Consent** Aprobación del Padre O Tutor

In the event of an illness or injury, I hereby authorize school officials on my behalf to obtain emergency transportation and treatment. En caso de enfermedad o lastimadura, doy mi autorización para que el personal de la escuela obtenga el tratamiento de emergencia y transporte. **I understand the school does not assume any financial responsibility for medical care or ambulance transportation in case of emergency. A Student Accident Policy is available to all students for a minimal fee.** Comprendo que la escuela no asume responsabilidad financiera por cuidados médicos o transporte en ambulancia en caso de emergencia. Existe una póliza estudiantil de accidentes para todos los alumnos, por una tarifa minima. **My signature acknowledges that I understand anc agree with the consent information above and that the information provided is complete and accurate.** Mi firma indica que comprendo y estoy de acuerdo con el consentimiento anterior, además de que la información incluida es completa y correcta.

Signature of Parent/Guardian Firma del padre o tutor_________________________**Date** Fecha_______________

▶ **As a parent/guardian, I grant permission for my child to participate in Righturn.Club activities. I also grant permission to use/publish my childs photograph, video , quotes or written statements for Righturn.Club promotional purposes.** Como padre/quarda, concedo el permiso para que la persona arriba nombrada participe en actividades del Righturn.Club. También concedo permiso para usar/publicar la persona fotografias, video, expresiones o declaraciones escritas de mi hijo o para los propósitos promocionales de Righturn.Club.

▶ **I,__________________________ (parent/legal guardian) hereby concent to the use of my childs oral and written statements and the use of their photograph(s) by Righturn.Club Mentoring Program.** Yo el padre/tutor) consiento por este medio el uso de las declaraciones orales y escritas de mi hijo/hija y el uso de sus fotografias por el programa de la tutoria de Righturn.Club.

▶ **I hereby release Righturn.Club and Kiwanis Club, and its agents and employees, from all claims, demands, liabilities whatsoever in connection with the above concent.** Libero por este medio el Righturn.Club and Kiwanis Club, y sus agentes y empleados, todas las reclamaciones, las demandas, responsabilidades cualesquiera que sean con respecto al consentimiento antes dicho.

Signature of Parent/Guardian Firma del padre o tutor_________________________**Date** Fecha_______________

▶ **Questions?** ¿Preguntas?____

____

Please return to school office when completed. Por favor regrese a la oficina de la escuela cuando esté terminado.

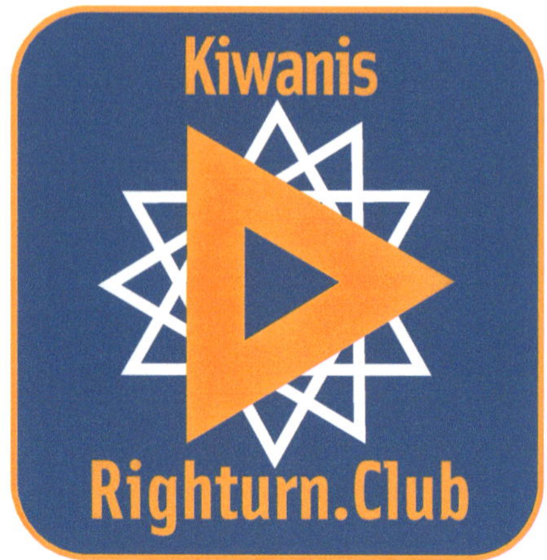

APPLICATION

School:_____________________

Time:_____________________

Dates:_____________________

Righturn.Club Mentor Information
Volunteer for 2 to 20 meetings

Last Name _____________________**First Name** _____________________**Middle Name** _____________________

Name of School You Are Interested In_____________________ **Date of Birth**_____________________

Home Street Address _____________________**City, State, Zip** _____________________

Home Telephone _____________________**Cell Phone** _____________________

Email _____________________**Prefered Method of Contact**_____________________

Educational Background: Name of School, Dates Attended, Diploma/Degree_____________________

____

____

Employment History: Name of Company, Position, Dates Worked, Employers for the last three years: _____________________

____

____

____

Community Service: Agency, Position, Dates Volunteered_____________________

____

____

____

Availability for Righturn.Club: Enter days of week available, and if you can give 2 hours each day for 10 weeks:

____

Preferred Days Check all the days you are available to volunteer:

☐ Monday ☐ Tuesday ☐ Wednesday ☐ Thursday ☐ Friday

☐ Monday & Wednesday ☐ Tuesday & Thursday ☐ Wednesday & Friday

Are you a student? _____________________

What months are you available?_____________________

You will be required to be fingerprinted at a local police station prior to start date. Are you willing to do this?_____________________

Can you speak/write in another language? How fluent?_____________________

Do you anticipate any changes in the next year that may interfere with your ability to Volunteer? _____________________

_____________________ **Please Complete Other Side**

▶ Health Information. Please complete the health information below. Check all that apply and describe.

___ Allergies, Include Type, food, bee, etc.____

___ Asthma ____

___ Diabetes ____

___ Heart Problem ____

___ Hemophilia ____

___ Other Health Concerns ____

▶ If you are under 18: Parent/Guardian Consent

In the event of an illness or injury, I hereby authorize school officials on my behalf to obtain emergency transportation and treatment. I understand the school does not assume any financial responsibility for medical care or ambulance transportation in case of emergency. A Student Accident Policy is available to all students for a mominal fee. My signature acknowledges tha I understand and agree with the consent information above and that the information provided is complete and accurate.

Signature of Parent/Guardian ____Date _____________________

As a parent/guardian, I grant permission for my child to participate in Righturn.Club activities. I also grant permission to use/publish my childs photograph, video , quotes or written statements for Righturn.Club promotional purposes.

▶ I,_______________________________ (parent/legal guardian) hereby concent to the use of my childs oral and written statements and the use of their photograph(s) by Righturn.Club Mentoring Program. I hereby release Righturn.Club and Kiwanis Club, and its agents and employees, from all claims, demands, liabilities whatsoever in connection with the above concent.

Signature of Parent/Guardian ____Date _____________________

▶ If you are an adult: My Consent

In the event of an illness or injury, I hereby authorize school officials on my behalf to obtain emergency transportation and treatment. I understand the school does not assume any financial responsibility for medical care or ambulance transportation in case of emergency. My signature acknowledges that I understand and agree with the consent information above and that the information provided is complete and accurate.

My Signature ____Date _____________________

▶ I grant permission to use/publish my photograph, video , quotes or written statements for Righturn.Club promotional purposes.

I,_______________________________ (Your Name) hereby concent to the use of my oral and written statements and the use of my photograph(s) by Righturn.Club Mentoring Program. I hereby release Righturn.Club and Kiwanis Club, and its agents and employees, from all claims, demands, liabilities whatsoever in connection with the above concent.

My Signature ____Date _____________________

Please return to school office when completed.

CHAPTER 4

Lesson Plans for 20 Meetings: Activity 1-20

The following pages are actual lesson plans used for each meeting. The general topics of health and fitness are covered each week. There is *flexibility* so that you can adjust them to your particular situation. They will be refered to as Activities. There are items to purchase, a list appears separately, that are used mostly more than once. The school would normally provide a way to show a video or play a song. Sound system equipment is not in the budget.

One mentor can effectively lead up to 20 children. The oldest children can be paired with the youngest to offset a lack of volunteers.

Some of our volunteers were high school students who only came for one hour, 3:15 to 4:15, when their schools ended. Elementary schools ended at 2:15, so from 2:15 to 3:15, the kids made their own snacks and drinks under supervision. Be very careful with knifes if cutting is involved.

You can also do a warmup with Salsa, Rock or other music and not follow a video choreo-graphed dance. You can improvise and just move, run in place, but have fun rather than engaging a formal push-up or calisthenic.

It's important to laugh and have fun, so lighten up and make the time with the kids very posi-tive and enjoyable. Teach one important rule: One person talks at a time, respecting everyone.

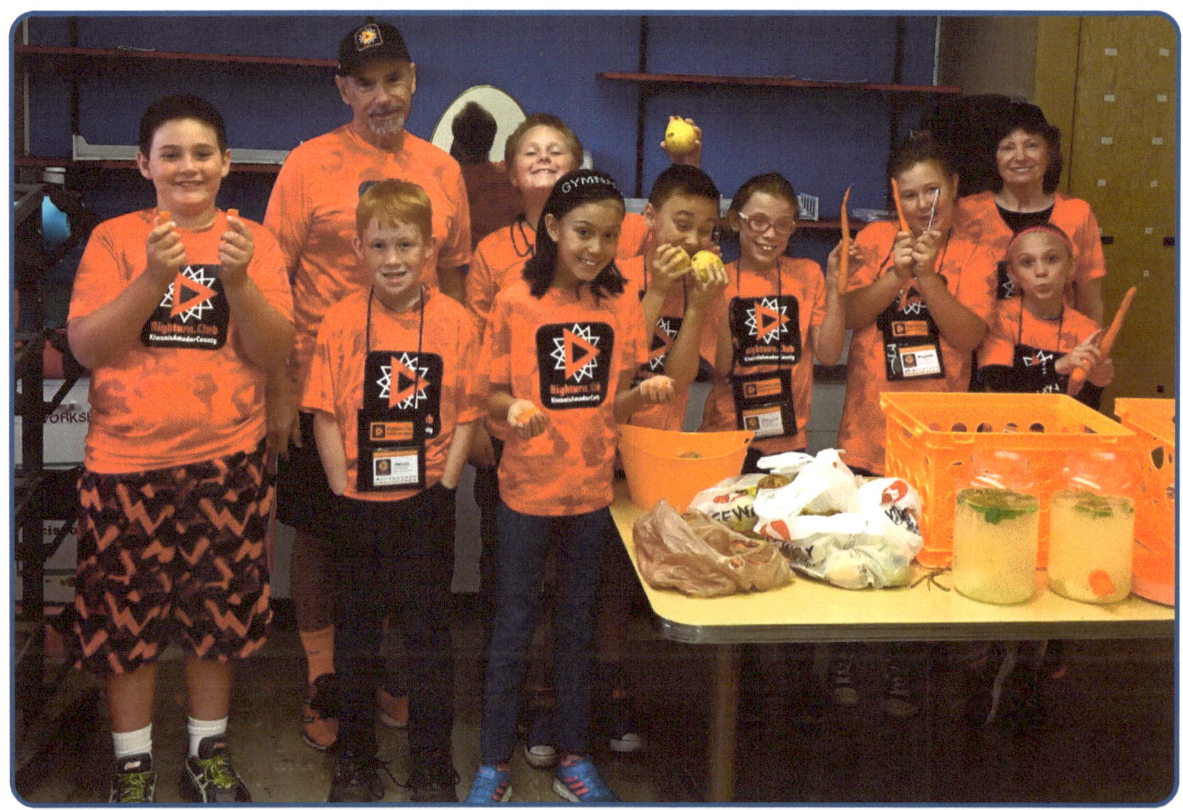

Kiwanis Rightturn.Club Kids at Sutter Creek Elementary School, Fall 2016. Mentor Roberta Ross helped greatly with the chats on nutrition. They prepared healthy snacks with some supervision.

Activity 1: Right Start—Get Ready to Rumble!

- Introduction of Members, Mentors and Guests
- Distribute Righturn.Club Shirt, Name Badge
- Complete Fitness and Nutrition Assessment-1
- Complete One Mile Timed Run
- Enjoy Snack and Infused Water
- Learn Memory Madness Game
- Learn Yoga Pose # 1 Upward Hand Pose: Standing, Arms stretched V

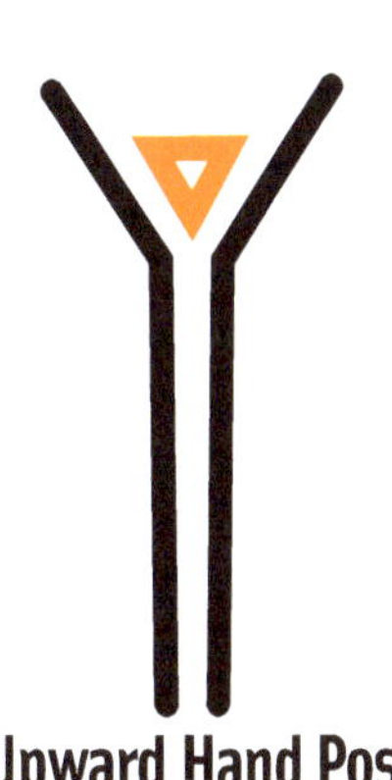

Upward Hand Pose

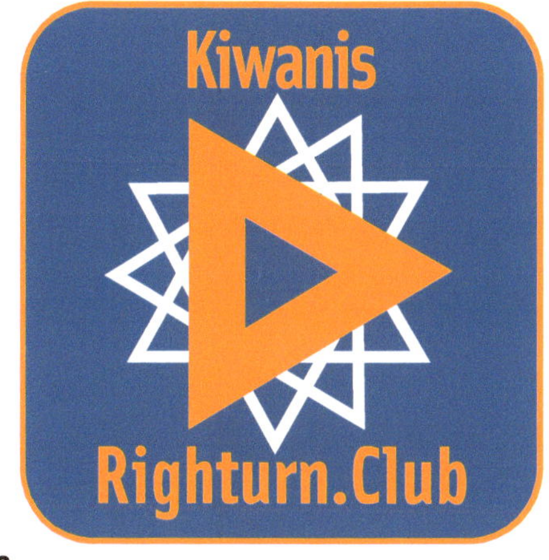

On Your Mark! 40 minutes

- **Healthy Snack and Drink Preparation**

Under supervision, kids will prepare healthy snack and prepare infused water drink. See suggestions in Chapter 5. Your local food bank may provide healthy fruits and veggies.

- Introductions of staff.
- Pass out shirts and badges.
- Take measurements, weight, hight, calculate BMI.
- **Fitness Chat Question:** What is Righturn.Club?

A: Righturn.Club is a mentor led fitness program that meets 2 times a week, members meet with a mentor. We will have fun and learn about healthy eating, how to lose extra weight and stay fit.

1. Righturn.Club T-shirt
   a. Wash every week.
   b. Bring and wear every meeting.
2. Righturn.Club Name Badge
   a. Wear for all activities
   b. Leave in basket and use at every meeting.

Get Set! 20 minutes

- **Take Fitness and Nutrition Assessment**

Members will complete a questionnaire today that will be repeated at the end of program.

- **Warm-up. Dance or Aerobic Movement to Music**

Go! 30 minutes

- **One Mile Run**
- **Healthy Snack and Water** Each member cleans up after themselves and the prep area.
- **Memory Madness Game** Stand in a circle.

Leader Says: "I'm going to Righturn.Club and I'm wearing my Righturn.Club T-Shirt. Yoga Pose # 1. Upward Hand Pose.

The next student says: "I'm going to Righturn.Club and I'm wearing my Righturn.Club T-Shirt and wearing running shoes. Strike pose # 1.

The second student says this and adds one more item. The members can add crazy imaginary items.

Items: Righturn.Club T-shirt, name badge, healthy snack, and infused water, paper plates and paper cups, scale, stopwatch (Cell Phone), tape measure, and *Fitness and Nutrition Assessment*.

Activity 2: Right Time—Just Go!

- Assign small group based on one mile run time and meet with mentor
- Introduce kids to correct running technique
- Warm-up: Play video and dance to Uptown Funk
- 1 mile run, water break at 1/2 mile mark
- Healthy snack and drink
- Play Memory Madness Game
- Learn Yoga Pose # 2 Tree 2 Pose Standing on one leg switch. Hands together

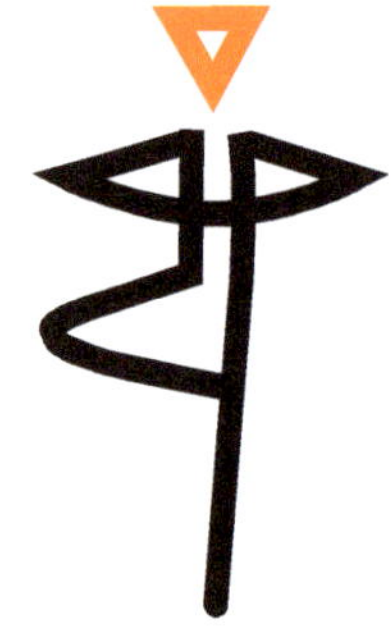

Tree 2

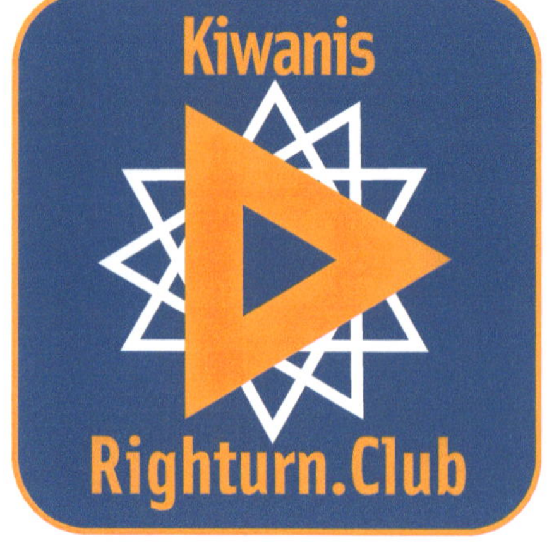

On Your Mark! 40 minutes

▶ Healthy Snack and Drink Preparation

Under supervision, kids will prepare healthy snack and prepare infused water drink. See suggestions in Chapter 5. Your local food bank may provide healthy fruits and veggies.

▶ Fitness Chat Question: Why should I run?

A: Running makes your body stronger, makes you feel better and helps to prevent disease.

1. Running makes your body stronger allover:
   - a. The heart is the most important muscle in the body and exercise makes it beat faster.
   - b. The more you run the more you build strength.
2. Running makes you feel better:
   - a. Running releases endorphins and helps make you happier.
   - b. Running with someone else encourages you and motivates you to push yourself further.
3. Running helps prevent diseases
   - a. Running helps prevent heart disease.
   - b. Running helps prevent diabetes.
   - c. Obesity
   - d. Depression

Get Set! 20 minutes

▶ Warm-up. Dance or Aerobic Movement to Music

Go! 30 minutes

▶ One Mile Run

Beforehand, in a car, determine route.

▶ Healthy Snack and Water

Each member cleans up after themselves and prep area.

▶ Memory Madness Game

Stand in a circle. Leader Says: "I'm going shopping for a healthy snack, and I'm buying some apples. Leader assumes Yoga Pose # 2. Tree Pose 2 One leg Balance, one leg on thigh. Switch. The next student says: "I'm going shopping for a healthy snack and I'm getting some apples and some oranges. Strike pose # 2. The second student says this and adds one more item. The members can add crazy imaginary items.

▶ Items Needed

Righturn.Club T-shirt, Name Badge, Healthy snack (Fruit/Veggies) and infused water, Paper plates and paper cups. For kids starting after the first meeting, have them do the timed run and Fitness/Nutrition Assessment 1.

Activity 3: Right Amount—Eat Halfsies!

▶ Learn about portion control and how to apply this at mealtime
▶ Introduce kids to eating half of portions
▶ Kids will apply what they learned about eating half a portion
▶ 1 mile run, water break at 1/2 mile mark
▶ Healthy snack and drink
▶ Play Memory Madness Game
▶ Learn Yoga Pose #3 Warrior Pose 1: Lunge, Arms Straight Up

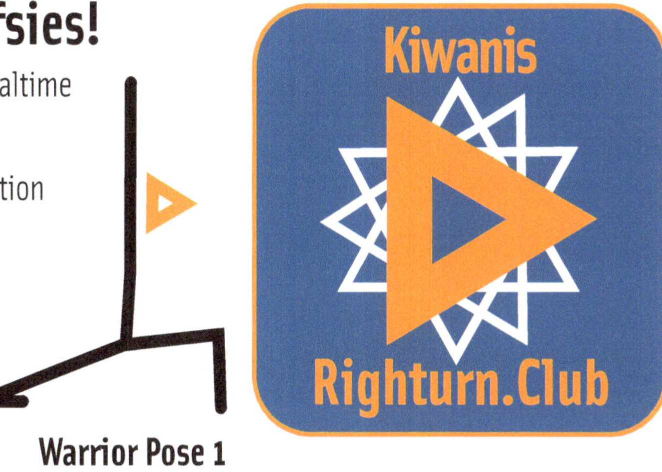

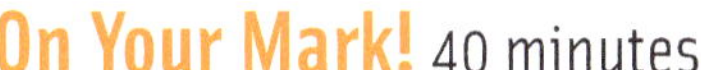
Warrior Pose 1

On Your Mark! 40 minutes

▶ **Healthy Snack and Drink Preparation**

Under supervision, kids will prepare healthy snack and prepare infused water drink. See suggestions in Chapter 5. Your local food bank may provide healthy fruits and veggies.

▶ **Nutrition Chat Question:** Why should I eat Halfsies? A: Reduces calories. Full portions are often more than your body needs. Helps you save money.

1. Reduces calories

    a. Calories are units of energy.

    b. The average person should consume the correct number of calories for you size.

    c. Eat the right amount for your size

2. Full portions are often more than you need.

    a. Never super size anything or order large.

    b. Eating slow helps you to enjoy your food more and eat less.

    c. Use a smaller plate or bowl when eating.

3. Helps you save money

    a. Have two meals for the price of one when eating out at a restaurant.

    b. Save half the food for another meal or snack.

Get Set! 20 minutes

▶ **Warm-up. Dance or Aerobic Movement to Music**

Go! 30 minutes

▶ **One Mile Run**

▶ **Healthy Snack and Water**

Each member cleans up after themselves and prep area.

▶ **Memory Madness Game** Stand in a circle. Leader Says: "Im going shopping for a healthy snack, and I'm buying some apples. Leader assumes Yoga Pose # 3. Warrior 1: Lunge, arms straight up.

The next student says: "I'm hungry for a healthy snack and I'm getting an apple. Strike pose # 3. The second student says this and adds one more item. The members can add crazy imaginary items.

▶ **Items Needed**

Righturn.Club T-shirt, name badge, healthy snack, and infused water, paper plates and paper cups.

For kids starting after the first meeting, have them do the timed run and *Fitness/Nutrition Assessment*, Eat Halfsies Magnets, tape measure and scale.

Optional but fun: Bring crazy sunglasses to wear.

Activity 4: Right Move—Friendly Running!

- Kids will learn that they will have more fun running side by side.
- Kids will walk, jog or run with a friend or family member this weekend for one hour.
- 2 mile run, Water break at 1 mile mark
- Healthy snack and drink
- Play Memory Madness Game
- Learn Yoga Pose # 4 Downward Facing Dog: Hands/Feet on floor.

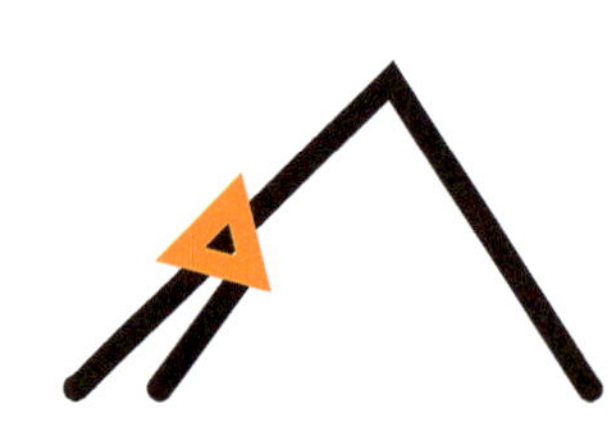

Downward Facing Dog

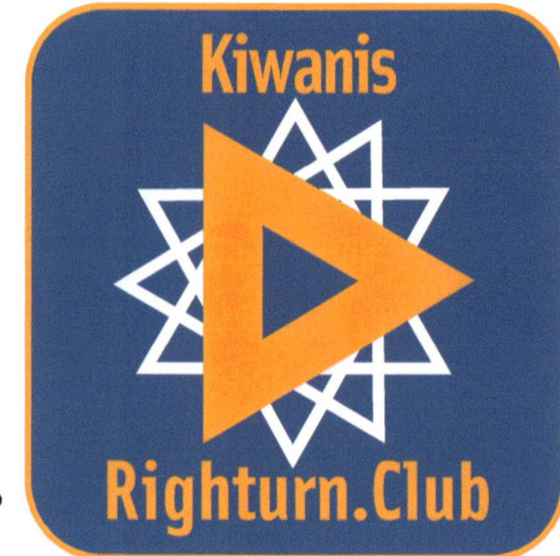

On Your Mark! 40 minutes

- **Healthy Snack and Drink Preparation**

Under supervision, kids will prepare healthy snack and prepare infused water drink. See suggestions in Chapter 5. Your local food bank may provide healthy fruits and veggies.

- **Fitness Chat Question:** Why should I run with a friend? A: Keeping up with each other helps you go faster and further. It also helps you make new friends.

1. Keeping up with each other helps you go further.
   a. Ask someone in your family or a friend at home to walk or run with you for one hour.
   b. Must be 1 hour or more.
2. Running with a friend will also help you make new friends. Be friendly.
   a. Going the distance with a friend is easier than going the distance alone.
   b. Making new friends is always a good thing.

Get Set! 20 minutes

- **Warm-up. Dance or Aerobic Movement to Music**

Go! 30 minutes

- **Two Mile Run** in Pairs
- **Healthy Snack and Water**

Each member cleans up after themselves and prep area.

- **Memory Madness Game** Stand in a circle. Leader Says: "I'm going for a run, and here's what I need to do. Set a time and day. Leader assumes Yoga Pose # 4. Downward Facing Dog. Hands/Feet on floor. The next student says: "I'm going for a run, and here's what I need to do. Set a time and day. Wear running Shoes. Strike pose # 4. The second student says this and adds one more item. The members can add crazy imaginary items.
- **Items Needed**

Righturn.Club T-shirt, name badge, healthy snack, and infused water, paper plates and paper cups, For kids starting after the first meeting, have them do the timed run and *Fitness/Nutrition Assessment* .

"Want friends? Be friendly." Thomas Moraitis

Activity 5: Right Drink—Water!

▶ Members will understand the value of water.

▶ They will make a choice to drink more water, at every meal

▶ 2 mile run, Water break at 1mile mark

▶ Healthy snack and drink

▶ Play Memory Madness Game

▶ Learn Yoga Pose # 5 Butterfly. Sitting,
   feet spread, hands together

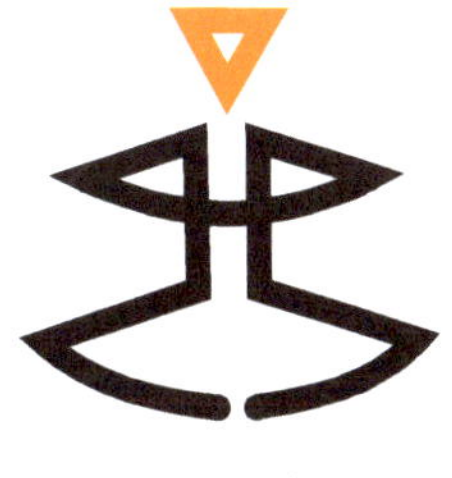

Butterfly 1

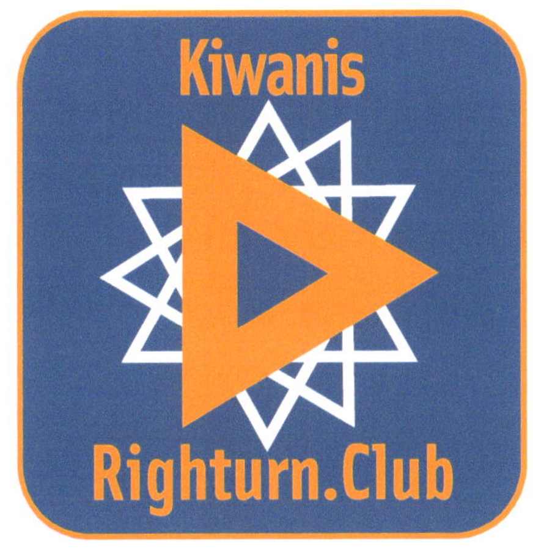

On Your Mark! 40 minutes

▶ **Healthy Snack and Drink Preparation**

Under supervision, kids will prepare healthy snack and prepare infused water drink. Your local food bank may provide healthy fruits and veggies.

▶ **Nutrition Chat Question:** Why should I drink water while running?

A: To balance body fluids and energize muscles. It makes your skin healthier. Drinking extra water can prevent dehydration.

1. Balance body fluids and energize muscles
    a. Water makes up more than half your weight.
    b. Each cell in your body depends on water to function normally.
2. Makes your skin healthier
    a. Water is very important for healthy skin
    b. Not enough water can make your skin look pale
3. Drinking extra water can prevent dehydration.
    a. Dilute any juice that you drink with water.
    b. Drink water before during and after your playing and or exercising.
    c. Drink extra water when it is hot outside.
4. Review the hydrology cycle
    a. Healthy Person = Healthy Planet
    b. Google hydrology for more fun facts.

▶ **Notes** Drinking water helps in weight loss. It can replace high calorie drinks. It's a great appetite suppressant. It contains no fat calories or carb's. It helps in making your heart healthier and lowers the risk of heart disease, headaches, cancer and skin problems. It also helps you digest your food better.

Get Set! 20 minutes

▶ **Warm-up. Dance or Aerobic Movement to Music**

Go! 30 minutes

▶ **Two Mile Run** in Pairs

▶ **Healthy Snack and Water**

Each member cleans up after themselves and prep area.

▶ **Memory Madness Game** Stand in a circle.

Leader Says: "I'm so thirsty. I'm going to drink water and not Coke. Leader assumes Yoga Pose # 5. Butterfly. On knees, feet spread hands together. The next student says: "I'm so thirsty, I'm going to drink water and not Coke or Pepsi. Strike pose # 5. The second student says this and adds one more item.

▶ **Items Needed**

Righturn.Club T-shirt, name badge, healthy snack, and infused water, paper plates and paper cups.

Activity 6: Right Track—New Healthy Habits!

- Kids will walk/jog/run with family members
- Kids will make a choice to do 60 minutes more, one day a week with a family member or friend.
- 2 mile run, Water break at 1mile mark
- Healthy snack and drink
- Play Memory Madness Game
- Learn Yoga Pose # 6 Cobra: On elbows, on floor, head up.

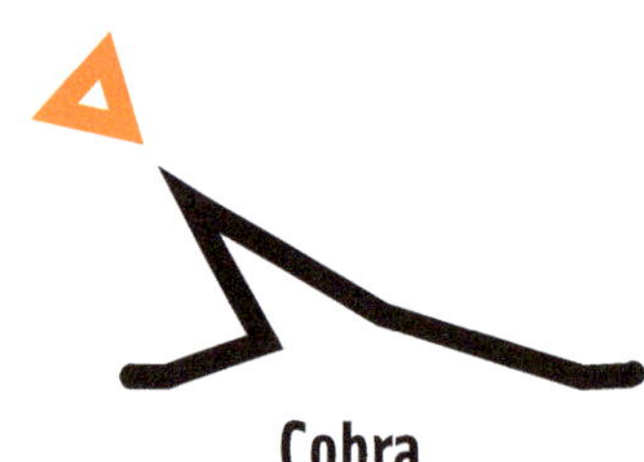

Cobra

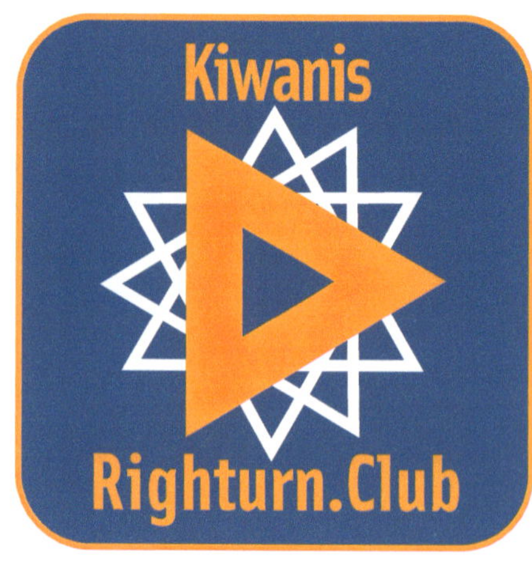

On Your Mark! 40 minutes

- **Healthy Snack and Drink Preparation**

Under supervision, kids will prepare healthy snack and prepare infused water drink. See suggestions in Chapter 5. Your local food bank may provide healthy fruits and veggies.

- **Fitness Chat Question:** Why should I get fit?

A: Fitness training helps you feel better physically and mentally. It provides one technique or approach to coping with emotional stress. It's the reason for getting fit that makes or breaks a healthy habit. It is a choice you can make and do something about it everyday.

1. Health benefits

    a. By just doing it we override being tired, depressed, bored, or feeling lazy.

    b. After starting and running, endorphins kick in and make you feel good

2. Just show up!

    a. Healthy intentions become healthy habits.

    b. Train at a certain day and time, don't be late.

Get Set! 20 minutes

- **Warm-up. Dance or Aerobic Movement to Music**

Go! 30 minutes

- **Two Mile Run** in Pairs
- **Healthy Snack and Water**

Each member cleans up after themselves and prep area.

- **Memory Madness Game** Stand in a circle.

Leader Says: "I want to go hiking and I'll bring comfy shoes. Leader assumes Yoga Pose # 6. Cobra: Elbows, on floor, head up. The next student says: "I want to go hiking and I'll bring comfy shoes and some water. Strike pose # 6. The second student says this and adds one more item. The members can add crazy imaginary items.

- **Items Needed**

Righturn.Club T-shirt, name badge, healthy snack, and infused water, paper plates and paper cups.

"Eat half, walk double, laugh triple and love without measure." Tibetan Proverb

Activity 7: Right Selection—Portion Control

▶ Members will learn that portion control is the key to eating healthy.

▶ They will learn that everyday items will help them remember the right amount to eat. Use activity sheet: Portion Patrol.

▶ Juggling lesson, then 2 mile run

▶ Healthy snack and drink

▶ Play Memory Madness Game

▶ Learn Yoga Pose # 7 Standing Bend: Feet on floor, hands on floor, look up.

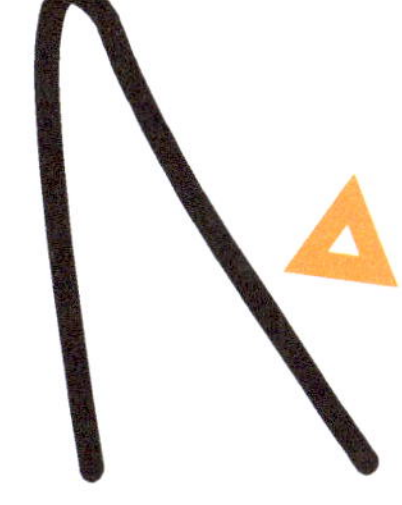

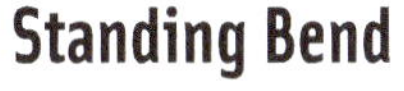

Standing Bend

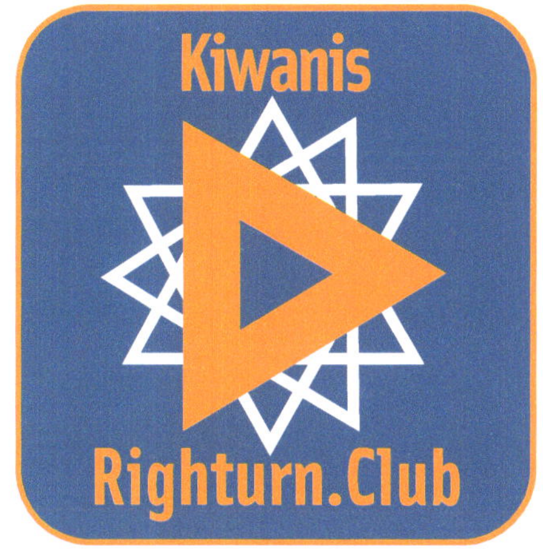

On Your Mark! 40 minutes

▶ **Healthy Snack and Drink Preparation**

Under supervision, kids will prepare healthy snack and prepare infused water drink. See suggestions in Chapter 5. Your local food bank may provide healthy fruits and veggies.

▶ **Nutrition Chat Question:** How can I be wise when it comes to size of portions?

A: Make foods look bigger by using a small salad plate or a small baggy. Only eat a handful of chips/pretzels not a bagful. Portion control is what will help you eat healthy.

1.Make food portions look bigger by using a small salad plate, bowl or baggy.

      a. This will help you eat the right size portion.

      b. You won't eat as much with a small plate instead of a large one.

2. Portion control items. Have each student hold them and give to next person.

      a. Deck of Cards = the size of meat, fish, or chicken, cake

      b. Golf Ball = the amount of peanut butter or nuts

      c. Baseball = the amount of rice, pasta, beans, potato, cereal, fruit

      d. AA Battery = the serving amount of cheese

      e. 1 Dice = the serving size of butter, dressing.

3. Eat as much vegetables as you want and eat small portions of other food.

Get Set! 20 minutes

▶ **Warm-up: How to Juggle Scarfs Lesson 1 of 3**

View or show You-Tube video on juggling scarfs.

Go! 30 minutes

▶ **Two Mile Run** in Pairs

▶ **Healthy Snack and Water**

Each member cleans up after themselves and prep area.

▶ **Memory Madness Game** Stand in a circle.

Leader Says: "I'm going out for dinner. I'm going to eat half the meat. Leader assumes Yoga Pose # 7. Standing Bend: Feet on floor, hands on floor, look up.

The next student says: "I'm going out for dinner. I'm going to eat half the meat and all the veggies. Strike pose # 7. The second student says this and adds one more item. The members can add crazy imaginary items.

▶ **Items Needed**

Righturn.Club T-shirt, name badge, healthy snack, and infused water, paper plates and paper cups, markers for handout. Scarves for juggling.

Activity 8: Right Beat–Cadence Running

▶ Kids will run stronger and faster and pace themselves by running while singing the Righturn.Club Cadence. Print out for each member.

▶ Members will learn the Righturn.Club Cadence

▶ Juggling Scarfs, Lesson 2, then 2 mile run

▶ Healthy snack and drink

▶ Play Memory Madness Game

▶ Learn Yoga Pose # 8 Boating Position: Balance on bottom, legs up arms straight.

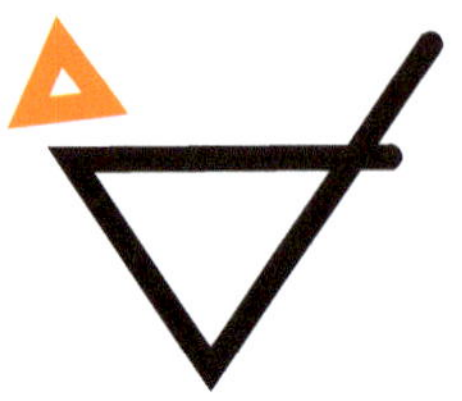

Boating Position

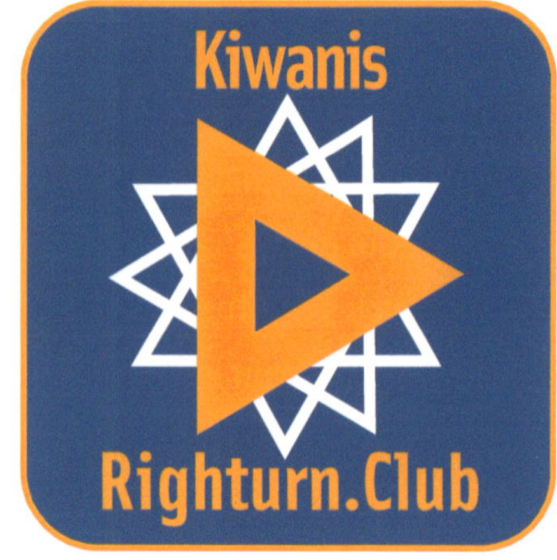

On Your Mark! 40 minutes

▶ **Healthy Snack and Drink Preparation**

▶ **Fitness Chat Question:** How can keeping the beat make me run faster?

A: Running to a cadence increases speed and endurance. Running to a cadence keeps you on pace and together.

Kiwanis Righturn.Club Cadence

Repeat all phrases. Short "Rights" are alphabetical

▶ **Righturn.Club you can't go wrong!**

▶ **Mentor led and going strong!**

▶ **All Right!**

▶ **Be Right!**

▶ **Do Right!**

▶ **Go Right!**

▶ **So Right!**

▶ **Join the club and have a ball!**

▶ **Righturn.Club is fun for all!**

Get Set! 20 minutes

▶ **Warm-up: How to Juggle Scarfs** Lesson 2. View or show U-Tube video on juggling scarfs.

Go! 30 minutes

▶ **Two Mile Run** in Pairs, Singing Cadence for beginning.

▶ **Healthy Snack and Water**

Each member cleans up after themselves and prep area.

▶ **Memory Madness Game** Stand in a circle.

Leader Says: "I'm going camping. I'm bringing a tent. Yoga Pose # 8 Boating Position: Balance on Bottom, legs up arms straight. The next student says: "I'm going camping. I'm bringing a tent and a flashlight. Yoga Pose # 8 Plank Position. The second student says this and adds one more item. The members can add crazy imaginary items.

▶ **Items Needed**

Righturn.Club T-shirt, name badge, healthy snack, and infused water, paper plates and paper cups, Cadence Cards, scarves for juggling. You can use plastic bags, too, for juggling.

"The heart beats fast, slow and normal, depending..." Thomas Moraitis

Activity 9: Right On—High Five!

▶ Help kids and parents eat five vegetables and fruits a day

▶ High Five Magnet will be given out

▶ They will record 5 days of eating five a day on handout

▶ Juggling Scarfs Lesson 3, then 2 mile run

▶ Healthy snack and drink

▶ Play Memory Madness Game

▶ Learn Yoga Pose # 9 Shoulder Stand: legs up, hold legs up with hands.

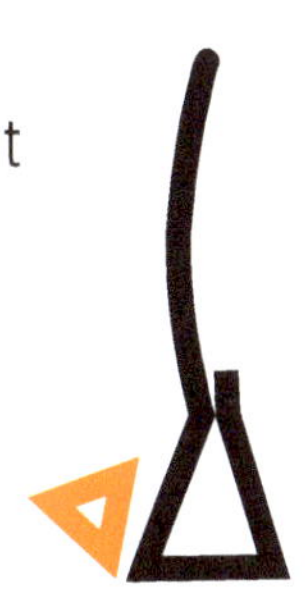
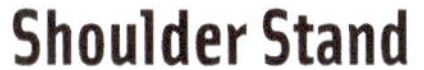

Shoulder Stand

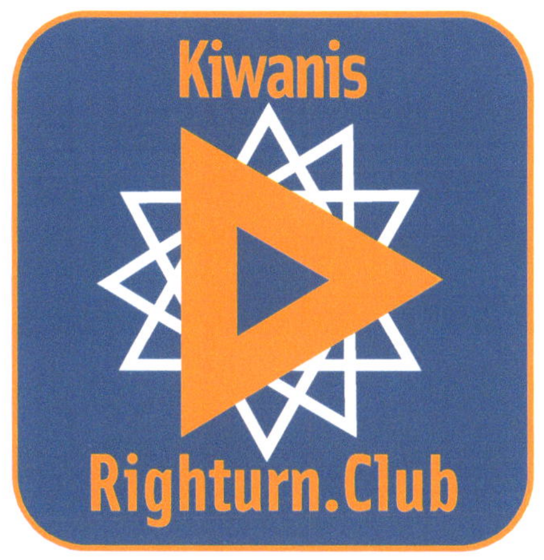

On Your Mark! 40 minutes

▶ **Healthy Snack and Drink Preparation**

▶ **Nutrition Chat Question:** Why should I eat 5 fruits and vegetables a day?

A: Eating fruits and vegetables is important for good health. It supports optimal growth, physical development, activity athletics, and learning. It helps prevent chronic diseases.

1. Fruits and vegetables are a good deal for both your health and for your wallet

   a. Healthy snacks like apples and carrots are cheaper than chips and donuts.

   b. Fruits and vegetables have vitamins and nutrients for healthier body's.

   c. Fruits and vegetables have less calories then candy and donuts.

2. Ask kids if they have a garden or if they'd like one.

   a. If they would like a garden in their home they can contact a local home garden club.

   b. They may have a school vegetable garden they could help with.

3. Generally speaking, the more colorful the vegetable the more nutritious.

Get Set! 20 minutes

▶ **Warm-up: How to Juggle Scarfs** Learn how to juggle Lesson 3. View or show You-Tube video on juggling.

Go! 30 minutes

▶ **Two Mile Run** in Pairs, Singing Cadence for beginning.

▶ **Healthy Snack and Water**

Each member cleans up after themselves and prep area.

▶ **Memory Madness Game** Stand in a circle.

Leader Says: "I'm going to start a garden. I'm planting carrots. Yoga Pose # 9 Shoulder Stand: legs up, hold legs up with hands. The next student says: "I'm going to start a garden. I'm planting carrots and tomatoes. Yoga Pose # 9 Sit cross legged. The second student says this and adds one more item. The members can add crazy imaginary items.

▶ **Items Needed**

Righturn.Club T-shirt, name badge, healthy snack, and infused water, paper plates and paper cups, scarves for juggling. High Five Magnets.High Five Handout.

Activity 10: Right Half—It's Half Time!

▶ Members will run a timed 1 mile.

▶ They will compare what they did at the start to this time.

▶ Healthy snack and drink

▶ Play Memory Madness Game

▶ Learn Yoga Pose # 10. Lie at Rest: On back, hands to side.

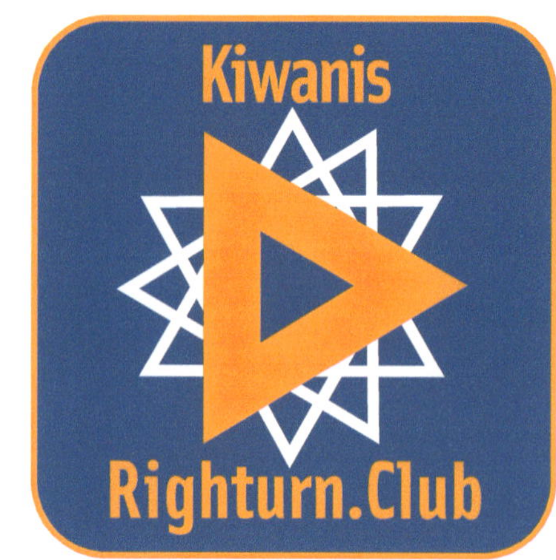

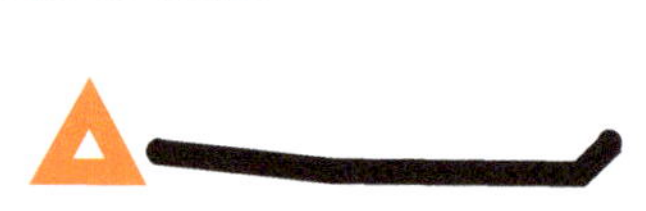

Lie and Rest

On Your Mark! 40 minutes

▶ **Healthy Snack and Drink Preparation**

▶ **Fitness Chat Question:** Why should I track my progress?

A: To see how much I've improved. It's good to see if you've made progress or not, then work harder to achieve more.

1. Keeping track of my results shows my progress.

    a. If my growth is slow then I need to push harder.

    b. Adjustments may need to be made.

Get Set! 20 minutes

▶ **Warm-up: Greek Dancing.** How to folk dance in a circle. Select from Greek, African or other nationality. Go to You-Tube and show video then dance along with the video. Pick a simple easy to follow dance. Suggestions. African Funga Dance. Greek Zorba Dance.

Go! 30 minutes

▶ **Two Mile Run** in Pairs

▶ **Healthy Snack and Water**

Each member cleans up after themselves and prep area.

▶ **Memory Madness Game** Stand in a circle. Leader Says: "I'm going to a football game. I'm bringing some healthy snacks. Yoga Pose # 10: Lie at Rest: On back, hands to side, facing up.

The next student says: "I'm going to a football game. I'm bringing some healthy snacks and a candy bar. Yoga Pose # 10. The second student says this and adds one more item. The members can add crazy imaginary items.

▶ **Items Needed**

Righturn.Club T-shirt, name badge, healthy snack, and infused water, paper plates and paper cups, video from YouTube on a Folk Dance.

"Believe you can and you're half way there."
Theodore Roosevelt

Activity 11: Right Choice—Right or Wrong Fat?

▶ Members will learn about the different kinds of fat

▶ They will read labels and limit bad fats

▶ At a fast food restaurant, they will choose not to supersize

▶ Healthy snack and drink

▶ Play Memory Madness Game

▶ Learn Yoga Pose # 11. Cow Position: On all fours, back down, head up

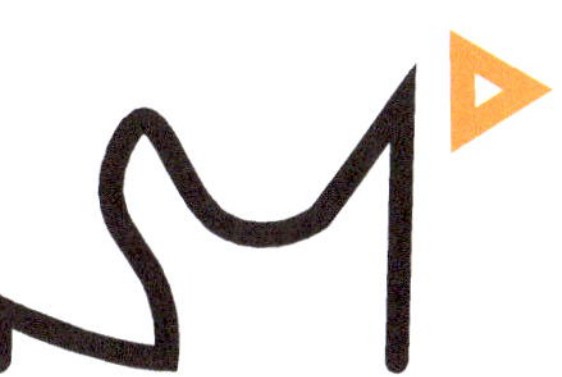

Cow Position

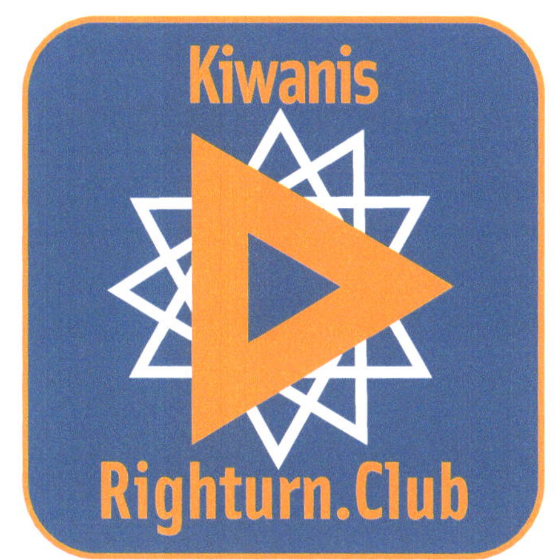

On Your Mark! 40 minutes

▶ **Healthy Snack and Drink Preparation**

▶ **Nutrition Chat Question:** How will I know which fats are right and which are wrong?

A: Read the labels. Learn the facts.

▶ **Skit: Mr. Wrong Fat and Mrs. Right Fat** No dialogue. Mr. Wrong Fat eats a huge donut, breaks it in half when kids say halfsies. Mrs. Right Fat eats some almonds with dried fruit or banana.

1. Right Fats: Unsaturated fats. Plant sources
    a. Raises your level of good cholesterol
    b. They contain antioxidants which are good .
    Examples: Fish oil and peanut butter, avocados
2. Polly-Unsaturated Fats: Polly = many
    a. Does not effect cholesterol levels
3. Wrong fats: Saturated fats. Animal sources
    a. These have high cholesterol levels
    b. This is found in packaged and fast food.
    Examples: Donuts, potato chips, cookies

▶ **Note:** Ask the kids to start reading labels. You don't know what kind of fat it is until you read the label.

Get Set! 20 minutes

▶ **Warm-up: Balloon Fun.** Balloon Fun: Fill 144 balloons with air, divide members in 2 teams: Right Fat and Wrong Fat. Right Fat sits and bursts ballons. Wrong Fat keeps them up in the air. See who wins.

Go! 30 minutes

▶ **Two Mile Run** in Pairs

Members will use Righturn Cadence to keep pace.

▶ **Healthy Snack and Water**

Each member cleans up after themselves and prep area.

▶ **Memory Madness Game** Stand in a circle.

Leader Says: "I'm going to buy snacks for movie night at my house. I'm buying bananas. Yoga Pose # 11. Cow Position: On all fours, back down, head up. The next student says: "I'm going to buy snacks for movie night at my house. I'm buying bananas and grapes. Yoga Pose # 11. The second student says this and adds one more item. The members can add crazy imaginary items.

▶ **Items Needed**

Righturn.Club T-shirt, name badge, healthy snack, and infused water, paper plates and paper cups, donut, and banana for skit, snack with label, 144 balloons.

Activity 12: Right Way—Game Day!

▶ Kids will learn about community fun runs.

▶ If there are no fun runs, 5 or 10 K's, do your own and invite parents and friends to come.

▶ Play Giant Tic-Tac-Toe Game, See drawing. Use 1-4

▶ Healthy snack and drink, Play Memory Madness Game

▶ Learn Yoga Pose # 12. Side Angle, Legs apart.

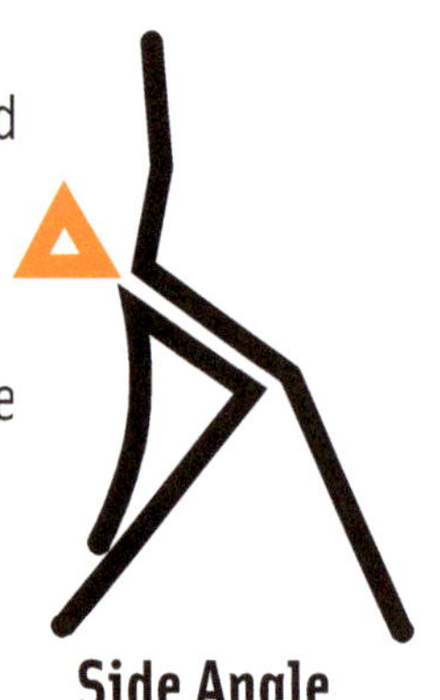

Side Angle

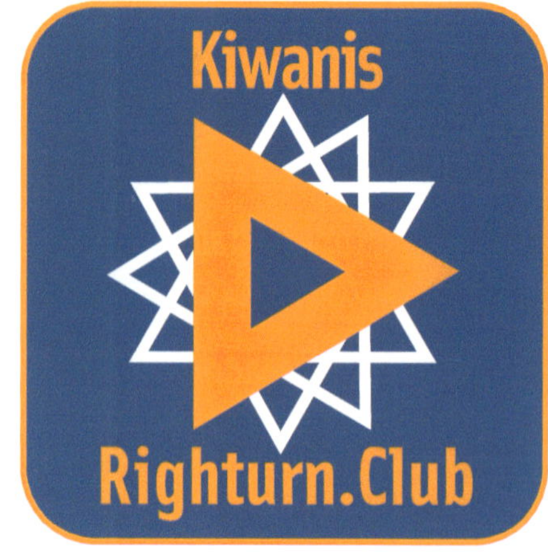

On Your Mark! 40 minutes

▶ **Healthy Snack and Drink Preparation**

▶ **Fitness Chat Question:** Why should I enter a fun run?

A: Its fun and I can see how fast I can run compared to other kids and adults.

1. Fun runs are timed

    a. You can see how you did.

2. Great Community events

    a. Parents are welcome to attend.

3. Being part of a group is emotionally rewarding

Get Set! 20 minutes

▶ **Warm-up: Tic-Tac-Toe Relay** See Illustration below. Divide kids into 2-4 groups with two teams each group. Kids race 25 yds from starting line to grid, placing a color square, then return. Next kid drops another square trying for acrosss, diagonal or down 3 in a row win.

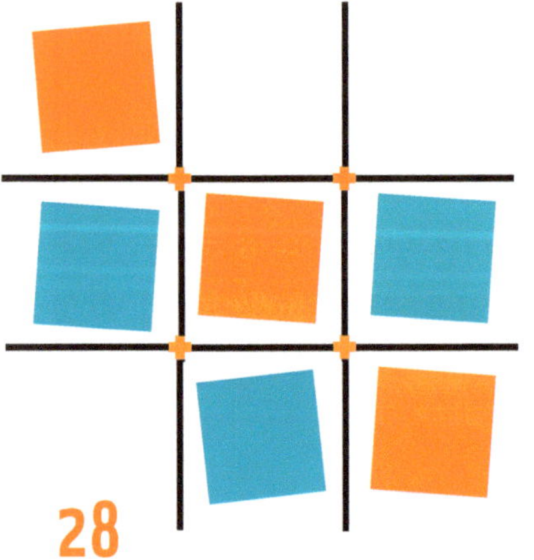

Each Tic-Tac-Toe Grid: 4-6 Players, 2-3 on a Team. 12, 2 ft White PVC Pipes and 4 Connectors with 3 contrasting color squares for each team.

Go! 30 minutes

▶ **Two Mile Run** in Pairs

▶ **Healthy Snack and Water**

Each member cleans up after themselves and prep area.

▶ **Memory Madness Game** Stand in a circle.

Leader Says: "I'm going to the toy store to buy a new game, and I'm going to get a big ball. Yoga Pose # 12. Plank: Like a push up, only up. The next student says: "I'm going to the toy store to buy a new game, and I'm going to get a big ball, and a frisbee. Yoga Pose # 12. The second student says this and adds one more item.

▶ **Items Needed**

For Tic=Tac-Toe Game: white PVC pipes and connectors, blanket squares.

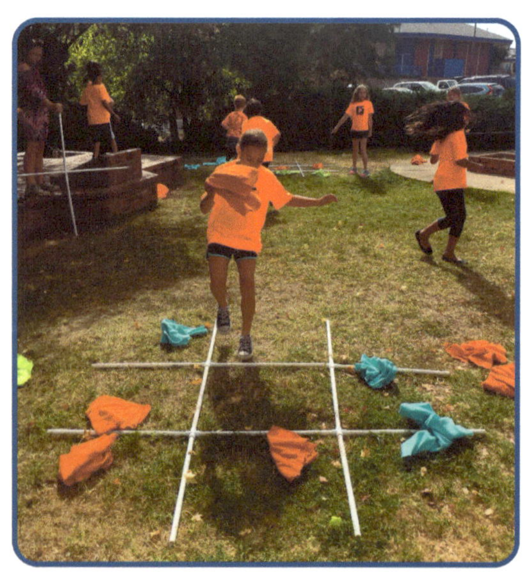

Fall 2017 at Sutter Creek Elementary School in Sutter Creek California

Activity 13: Right Thing—Protein Hunting!

▶ Members will learn about why their body needs protein.

▶ They will be able to identify high protein food items.

▶ Play Protein Cone Relay

▶ Healthy snack and drink

▶ Play Memory Madness Game

▶ Learn Yoga Pose # 13. Standing Bow: On one leg, one hand straight, the other holding foot.

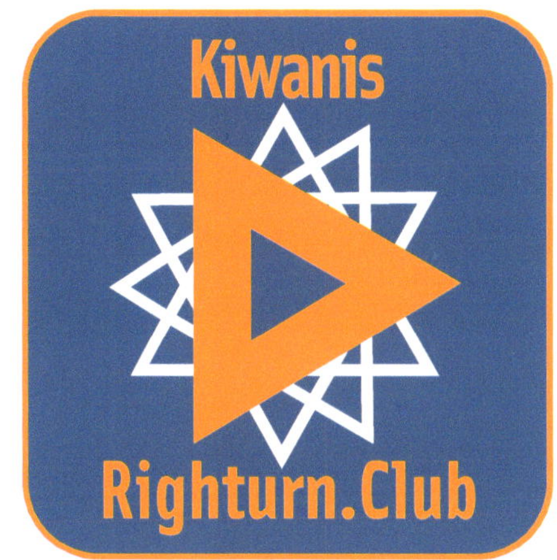

Standing Bow

On Your Mark! 40 minutes

▶ **Healthy Snack and Drink Preparation**

▶ **Nutrition Chat Question:** Why does my body need protein? Is it hard to find?

A: Protein helps build and repair muscles and gives me energy. It's found abundantly in meat, chicken and fish. Eggs, peanut butter, cheese, soy and nuts are also good.

1. Helps build strong muscles and bones

    a. Food with protein helps you feel less hungry

    b. You can run further with some protein, like a peanut snack.

2. Foods that are good sources of protein are:

    a. Meat, chicken, fish, low fat cheese, eggs, peanut better,nuts and seeds.

Get Set! 20 minutes

▶ **Warm-up: Protein Cone Relay**

Members will run from cone to cone and write on *My Turn Card* a list of 12 items. Each cone will have an activity, and a letter. The letter will make up a surprise phrase to do with protein-BUILDS MUSCLE. The kids don't have to go in any order, but need to go to every cone and get there by circling the center marker. Place 12 cones around a grassy field in a very large circle.

1. Name a dairy food high in protein.

2. Name a breakfast food high in protein.

3. Name a beverage high in protein.

4. Name a meat high in protein.

5. Name a seafood high in protein.

6. Name a poultry food high in protein.

7. Name a canned food high in protein.

8. Name a deli food high in protein.

9. Name a snack high in protein.

10. Name a nut product high in protein.

11. Name a vegetable high in protein.

12. Name your all-time favorite high protein food.

Go! 30 minutes

▶ **Two Mile Run** in Pairs

▶ **Healthy Snack and Water**

Each member cleans up after themselves and prep area.

▶ **Memory Madness Game** Stand in a circle.

Leader Says: "I'm going to move more, and take walks. Yoga Pose # 13. Childs Pose. The next student says: "I'm going to move more, and take walks, ride my bike. Yoga Pose # 13. The second student says this and adds one more item.

The members can add crazy imaginary items.

▶ **Items Needed**

Righturn.Club T-shirt, name badge, healthy snack, and infused water, paper plates and paper cups, 12 orange cones, 1 large center cone, 12 strips of instruction.

Activity 14: Right Beat—My Heart Rate!

▶ Members will understand what interval training is.

▶ Members will learn how to take their own heart rate.

▶ Play Nutrition Treasure Hunt Relay

▶ Healthy snack and drink, play Memory Madness Game

▶ Learn Yoga Pose # 14. Easy Pose: Sitting, knees apart, hands on knees.

▶ Kids will listen to their heart with stethoscopes.

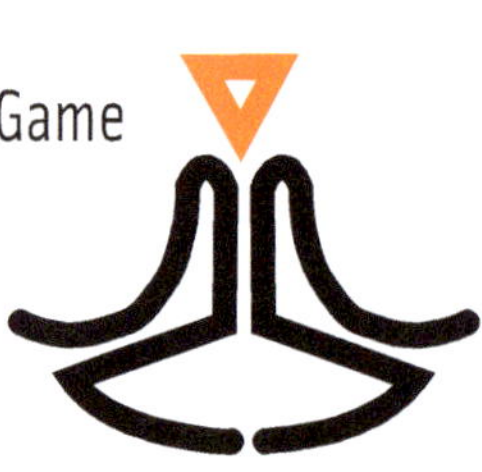

Easy Pose

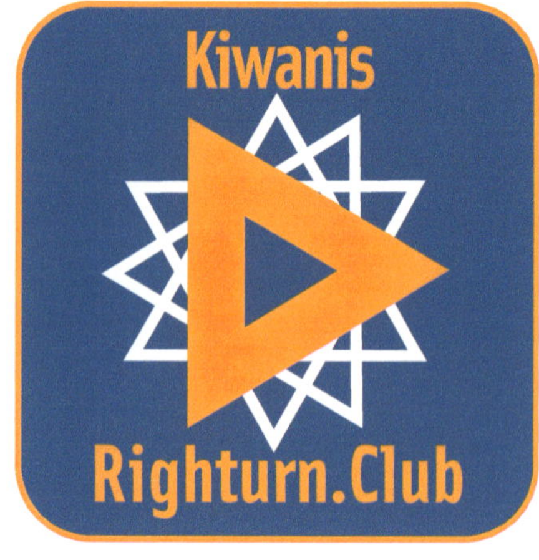

On Your Mark! 40 minutes

▶ **Healthy Snack and Drink Preparation**

▶ **Nutrition Chat Question:** What is my heart rate sitting? What is my heart rate after running in place for 3 minutes?

The faster your heart beats the more oxygen you get. Varying pace improves endurance.

1. The heart is the most important muscle in the body.

    a. When the heart becomes stronger it pumps more blood.

2. The more you train the stronger your heart becomes,

    a. The more you train the less tired you feel.

Get Set! 20 minutes

▶ **Warm-up: Nutrition Cone Relay**

Members will run from cone to cone and write on *My Turn Card* a list of 12 items. Each cone will have an activity, and a letter. The letter will make up a surprise phrase to do with nutrition-RIGHTURN CLUB. The Members don't have to go in any order, but need to go to every cone and get there by circling the center marker. Place 12 cones around a grassy field in a very large circle.

1. Name something to eat using halfsies.

2. Name something to eat that is a right fat or good fat.

3. Name something to eat that is a wrong fat or bad fat.

4. What is the right portion for the size of cheese?

5. What is the right portion for the size of meat?

6. What is the right portion for the size of veggies?

7. What should you wear to Righturn.Club?

8. Why should you run with a friend?

9. Why should you eat protein everyday?

10. Why should you avoid drinking soda?

11. What have you learned at Righturn.Club that changed the way you eat?

12. What is your favorite game or activity?

Go! 30 minutes

▶ **Two Mile Run** on Track

Track interval training: Run straightways, walk curves.

▶ **Healthy Snack and Water**

Each member cleans up after themselves and prep area.

▶ **Memory Madness Game** Stand in a circle. Leader Says: "I'm going to eat healthy and eat halfsies. Yoga Pose # 14. Standing Fold. The next student says: "I'm going to eat healthy and eat halfsies, only a handful of chips. Yoga Pose # 14. The second student says this and adds one more item. The members can add crazy imaginary items.

▶ **Items Needed**

Righturn.Club T-shirt, name badge, healthy snack, and infused water, paper plates and paper cups, 12 orange cones, 1 large center cone, 12 strips of instruction. See page 48, Stethoscopes.

Activity 15: Right Quantity—Carb's Fuel Energy

▶ Kids will learn to eat the right amount of carbohydrates.

▶ They will understand what a simple and complex carbohydrate is.

▶ Healthy snack and drink

▶ Play Memory Madness Game

▶ Learn Yoga Pose # 15. Cat Pose: On hands and knees, Back arched up.

Cat Pose

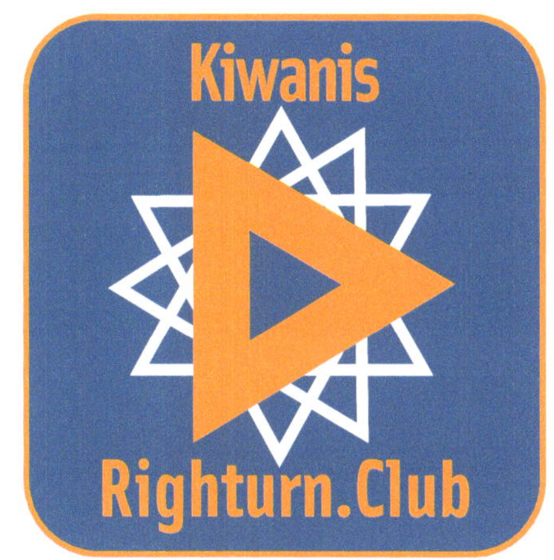

On Your Mark! 40 minutes

▶ **Healthy Snack and Drink Preparation**

▶ **Nutrition Chat Question:** What should I know about carbohydrates?

A: Carbohydrates are our main source of energy. There are two kinds of carbohydrates.

1. Two kinds of carbohydrates

    a. Complex carbohydrates.

    b. Simple carbohydrates.

2. Complex Carbohydrates

    a. Eat in larger portions

    b. Examples: Oatmeal, whole fruits and vegetables, brown rice, whole grain bread, beans, cucumber, lettuce

3. Simple Carbohydrates

    a. Eat less

    b. Examples: candy, sugar, fruit juices

4. These Carbohydrates should be chosen less often

    a. Potato chips, white rice, white bread, mashed potatoes, sugary breakfast food, candy, soda

Get Set! 20 minutes

▶ **Warm-up: Ping Pong Bounce**

Using ping pong balls and egg crates, divide the group into small groups of 4 each. Two on a team. Each team has 6 cards facing down. 2 colors of ping balls per table. Each team makes the formation on the cards. Winning teams play each other until a Champion Team has won.

Go! 30 minutes

▶ **Two Mile Run** in Pairs

Members run two miles on course.

▶ **Healthy Snack and Water**

Each member cleans up after themselves and prep area.

▶ **Memory Madness Game** Stand in a circle. Leader Says: "I'm going to the fair, and can't wait to eat corn on the cob. Yoga Pose # 15: Cat Pose. The next student says: "I'm going to the fair, and can't wait to eat corn on the cob and an apple. Yoga Pose # 15. The second student says this and adds one more item. The members can add crazy imaginary items.

▶ **Items Needed**

Righturn.Club T-shirt, name badge, healthy snack, and infused water, paper plates and paper cups, ping pong balls, egg crates, Ping Pong Bounce Cards.

Activity 16: Right Mind=Right Body & Choice

▶ Kids will learn to make healthy decisions for a healthy future

▶ They will make one change in adding more activity

▶ Healthy snack and drink

▶ Play Memory Madness Game

▶ Learn Yoga Pose # 16. Warrior Pose 2. Lunge, arms outstretched, face to side.

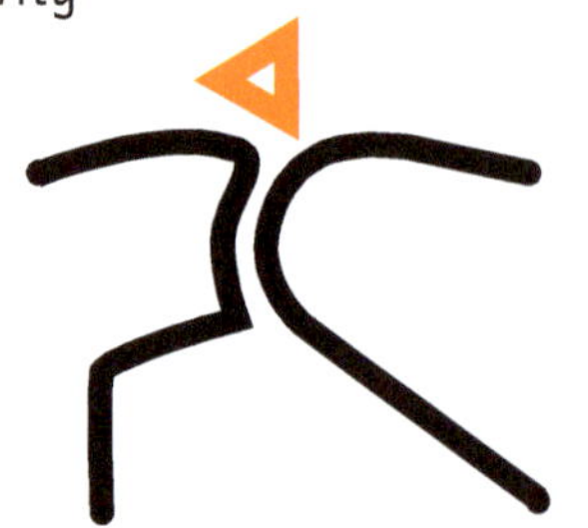

Warrior Pose 2

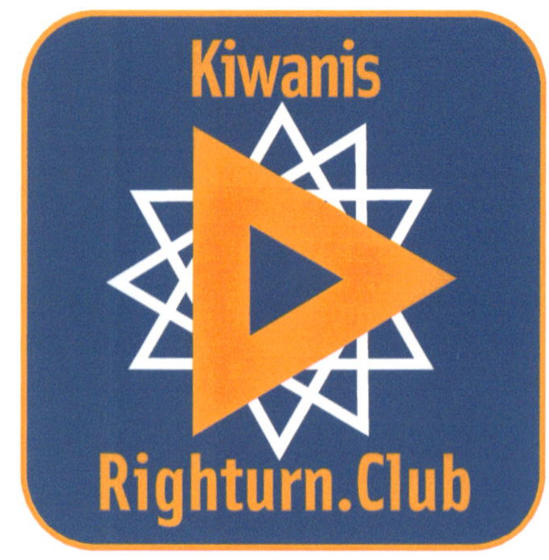

On Your Mark! 40 minutes

▶ **Healthy Snack and Drink Preparation**

▶ **Fitness Chat Question:** What choice can I make today that will impact my future?

A: Move more sit less. Discover your favorite activities.

1. Move more sit less

    a. Being active helps you do better in school.

    b. Being more active makes you less tired and bored.

    c. Being more active helps you feel better physically, emotionally and mentally.

2. Being more active:

    a. Can build your confidence

    b. Going the distance in running can help you go the distance in other things.

Get Set! 20 minutes

▶ **Warm-up: Beginning Yoga Practice**

We have learned various Yoga poses. Pick a Child's Yoga Video on YouTube and follow along. Or play quiet music, and lead a 20 minute sequence of poses. Pay special attention to the breath. Breathing in and out slowly and deeply.

Go! 30 minutes

▶ **Two Mile Run** in Pairs

Members run two miles on course.

▶ **Healthy Snack and Water**

Each member cleans up after themselves and prep area.

▶ **Memory Madness Game** Stand in a circle. Leader Says: "I'm going to be more active this vacation, and will ride my bike. Yoga Pose # 16: Warrior 2. The next student says: "I'm going to be more active this vacation, and will ride my bike, do some skating. Yoga Pose # 16. The second student says this and adds one more item. The kids can add crazy imaginary items.

▶ **Items Needed**

Righturn.Club T-shirt, name badge, healthy snack, and infused water, paper plates and paper cups, Yoga Video from YouTube.

"Even the smallest actions are steps in the right direction."

Activity 17: Right Side—Eat This, Not That!

- Kids will learn to make better choices on what to eat and what not to eat.
- They will make one change in their eating habits from "Eat This, Not That"
- They will learn the value of food swaps that can help them get fit, lose weight and eat healthy.
- Healthy snack and drink
- Play Memory Madness Game
- Learn Yoga Pose # 17. Seated Front Bend: Seated, legs & arms extended.

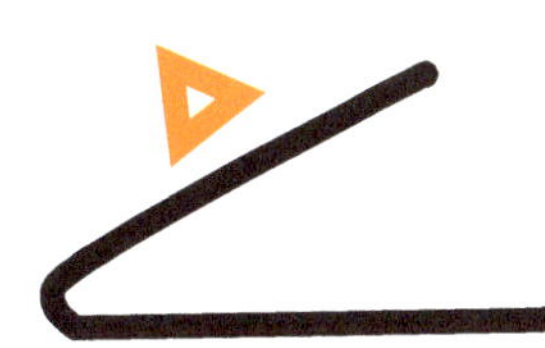

Seated Front Bend

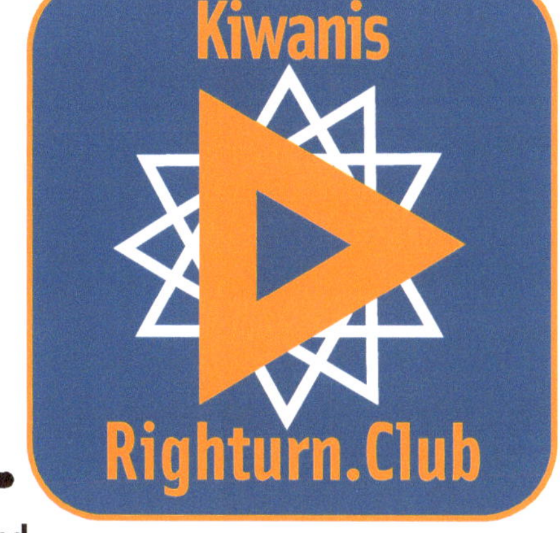

On Your Mark! 40 minutes

- **Healthy Snack and Drink Preparation**
- **Nutrition Chat Question:** Why should I choose to eat healthier foods?

A: Healthy choices will give you more energy and help you to stay fit.

1. Fast Foods

   a. Eat halfsies, like fries and hamburgers.

   b. Never supersize, never drink regular soda, instead choose juice, milk or water.

   c. Choose a fruit, salad or yogurt.

2. Restaurants or Family dinners:

   a. Ask for an extra plate or bowl and split meals

   b. No seconds.

   c. Don't do email, read or watch TV while eating.

3. At Home

   a. Eat one handful of chips

   b. Use a small salad plate or bowl

4. Nutrition Guides at Fast Food Restaurants

   a. All these places have them, so read them.

Get Set! 20 minutes

- **Warm-up: Beginning Yoga Practice**

We have learned various Yoga poses. Pick a Childs Yoga on YouTube and follow along. Or play quiet music, and lead a 20 minute sequence of poses. Pay special attention to the breath. Breathing in and out slowly and deeply.

Go! 30 minutes

- **Two Mile Run** in Pairs

Members run two miles on course.

- **Healthy Snack and Water**

Each member cleans up after themselves and prep area.

- **Memory Madness Game** Stand in a circle. Leader Says: "I'm going to eat less French Fries. Yoga Pose # 17: Seated Front Bend. The next student says: "I'm going to eat less French Fries and Fried Chicken. Yoga Pose # 17. The second student says this and adds one more item. The members can add crazy imaginary items.

- **Items Needed**

Righturn.Club T-shirt, name badge, healthy snack, and infused water, paper plates and paper cups, Yoga video from YouTube.

Activity 18: Right Advise—3 Corners of Fitness!

▶ Make a right turn to fitness: Get Ready, Get Set and GO!

▶ Kids will continue to run after the program is over.

▶ They will work out 2-3 times a week.

▶ Healthy snack and drink

▶ Play Memory Madness Game

▶ Learn Yoga Pose #18. Upward Bow: On Back knees bent, hands bent, then push up to extend arms and legs.

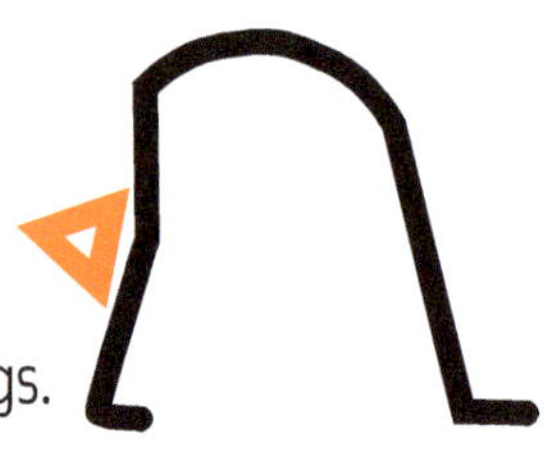

Upward Bow

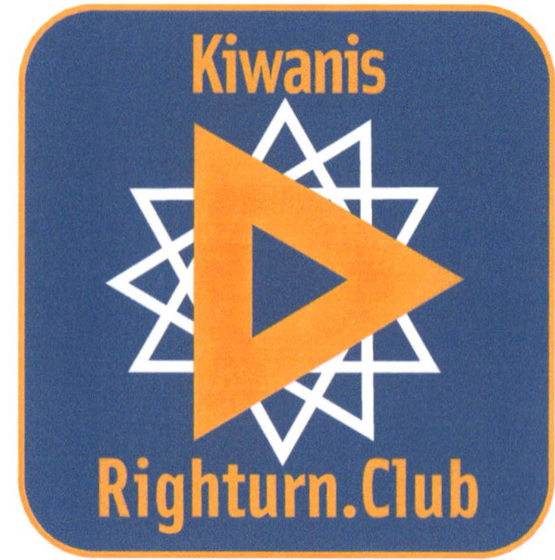

On Your Mark! 40 minutes

▶ **Healthy Snack and Drink Preparation**

▶ **Fitness Chat Question:** What are the 3 Corners of Fitness?

1. *Do it with Someone:* Friend or Family Member

2. *Have Fun:* Talk, Laugh and vary the activity

3. *Twice a week:* Try to keep to the schedule

    1. Do it with someone.

        a. Stop the excuses, prepare, and GO.

        b. Running makes your body stronger, makes you feel better and helps prevents diseases.

        c. Ask a friend or relative to meet you. That way you are more likely to do it.

    2.Have Fun.

        a. Wear silly clothes, joke around, laugh.

        b. Running with a friend helps you go further and faster and don't forget to have F U N.

    3. Twice a week.

        a. Decide which days and times you will go.

        b. Your health will improve by being more active two or three times a week.

Get Set! 20 minutes

▶ **Warm-up: Beginning Yoga Practice**

We have learned various Yoga poses. Pick a Childs Yoga Video on YouTube and follow along. Or play quiet music, and lead a 20 minute sequence of poses. Pay special attention to the breath. Breathing in and out slowly and deeply.

Go! 30 minutes

▶ **Two Mile Run** in Pairs

Members run two miles on course.

▶ **Healthy Snack and Water**

Each member cleans up after themselves and prep area.

▶ **Memory Madness Game** Stand in a circle. Leader Says: "I'm going to start biking and bring a friend. Yoga Pose # 18: Upward Blow. The next student says: "I'm going to start biking and bring a friend, wear a helmet. Yoga Pose # 18. The second student says this and adds one more item. The members can add crazy imaginary items.

▶ **Items Needed**

Righturn.Club T-shirt, name badge, healthy snack, and infused water, paper plates and paper cups, Yoga video from YouTube.

Activity 19: Right Purpose—3 Corners of Eating!

▶ Eat halfsies, limit portions and make wise food choices
▶ Members will make one change based on what they learned today when it comes to healthy eating.
▶ Healthy snack and drink
▶ Play Memory Madness Game
▶ Learn Yoga Pose # 19. Chathuranga: Push-up plank on elbows

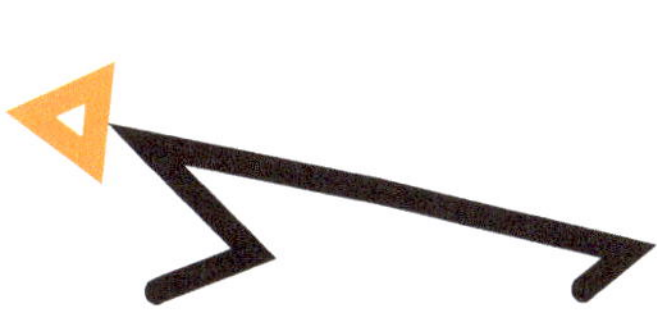

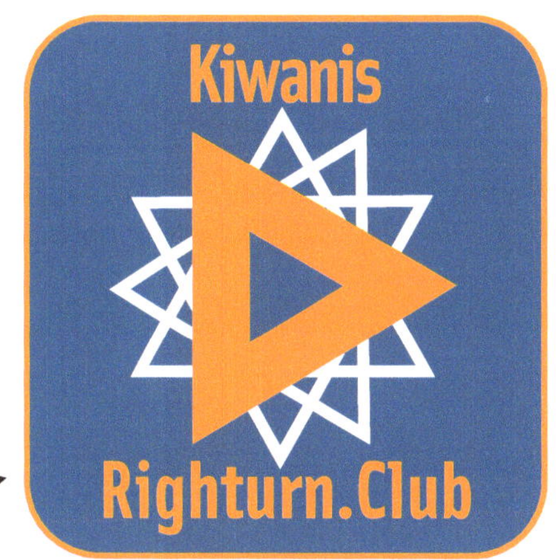

Chathuranga

On Your Mark! 40 minutes

▶ **Healthy Snack and Drink Preparation**

▶ **Nutrition Chat Question:** What are the 3 Corners of Healthy Eating?

1. *Right Choices*
2. *Right Portions*
3. *Right Balance*

   1. Right Choices

      a. Eat this, Not that kinds of choices.

      b. Don't supersize, choose small.

2. Right Portion

      a. Remember the size of portions: ball, golf ball, deck of cards, handful of chips, etc.

      b. Use a small salad plate or bowl

4. Right Balance

      a. Choose 5 fruits and vegetables a day.

      b. Choose to balance protein, carb's and fats

▶ **Take Post Test: My Statistics** On page 56

Get Set! 20 minutes

▶ **Warm-up: 4,3,2,1 Relay**

Place 12 cones in a large circle like a clock. The size of the circle will vary, but use a grassy area. The Members run one min. then walk one min. Change direction.

Next run 2 min., walk 2 min. Change direction. Next run 3 min., walk 3 min. Change direction. Finally run 4 min., walk 4 min.

Go! 30 minutes

▶ **Two Mile Run** in Pairs

Members run two miles on course.

▶ **Healthy Snack and Water**

Each member cleans up after themselves and prep area.

▶ **Memory Madness Game** Stand in a circle. Leader Says: "I'm going to a Fast Food Restaurant and ordering a small burger. # 19: Chathuranga. The next student says: "I'm going to a Fast Food Restaurant and ordering a small burger, a small fry. Yoga Pose # 19. The second student says this and adds one more item. The members can add crazy imaginary items.

▶ **Items Needed**

Righturn.Club T-shirt, name badge, healthy snack, and infused water, paper plates and paper cups, 12 orange cones, stopwatch.

Activity 20: Right Advise—Excel Still More!

▶ Kids will complete a timed one mile run.
▶ They will make a decision to continue with the lessons learned at Righturn.Club.
▶ Certificate of Excellence given to each participant.
▶ Healthy snack and drink with Family Members
▶ Play Balloon Toss
▶ Write Giving Thanks Cards and Righturn.Club is...
▶ Final weight and *Fitness and Nutrition Assessment*

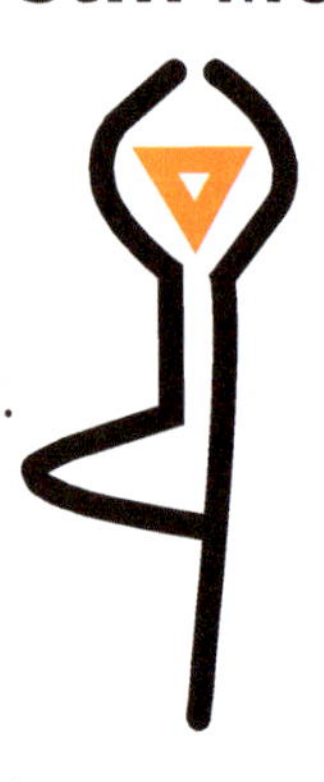

Tree 1

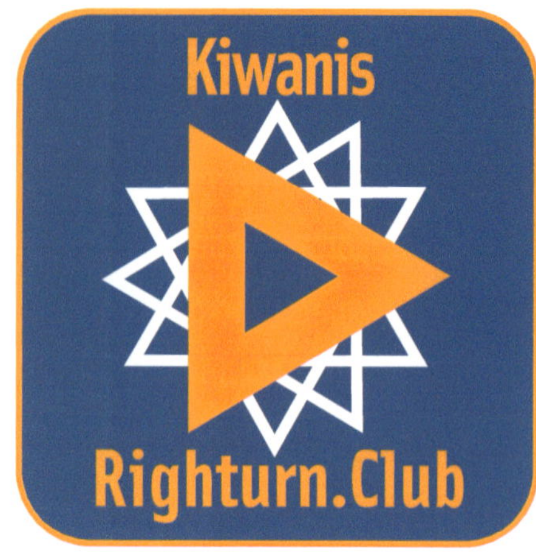

On Your Mark! 40 minutes

▶ **Healthy Snack and Drink Preparation**

▶ **Nutrition & Fitness Chat Question:** Why should I continue with Righturn.Club?

A: To help me make better food choices and be more active.

1. Timed 1 mile Run

    a. Encourage Members to push hard and do better than ever.

    b. Record on Chart

▶ **Giving Thanks Cards** Each student signs thank you cards that are given to all who helped during Righturn.Club.

▶ **Righturn.Club Is...** Cards Each student writes their thoughts and or what they learned in the last ten weeks.

Get Set! 20 minutes

▶ **Warm-up: Balloon Toss**

Divide into two facing teams, in pairs. Toss water balloon. Take a step back, repeat, Another step, repeat. If your balloon breaks, you are out.

Go! 30 minutes

▶ **One Mile Timed Run**

Members run one mile on track or course.

▶ **Certificate of Excellence**

Each member receives a framed award.

▶ **Healthy Snack and Water**

Each member cleans up after themselves and prep area.

▶ **Items Needed**

Righturn.Club T-shirt, name badge, healthy snack, and infused water, paper plates and paper cups, stopwatch, bathroom scale, certificates in plastic frames, Giving Thanks Cards, Righturn.Club... is Cards.

"Success is simple. Do what's right, the right way, at the right time." Arnold Glasow

CHAPTER 5

Healthy Snack Ideas

Kids love the unexpected, the unusual and treats. So to make what they eat and drink, fun, they are involved in the process. Our local food bank agreed to provide healthy snacks, but they always don't have everything you might need. So supplement with fresh fruits and vegetables as needed.

"Running is not hard. Just make sure you're running in the RIGHT direction."

Infused Water Beverage aka Agua Fresca

Use a very large container with a removable top and spigot. We used an orange container usually found at a Hardware store used for water. Do not serve soda--diet or regular, prepared sugary drinks or bottled water. Here are 12 suggested combinations to add to cool water. You may add ice. Bring tongs, to give fruit to kids after they drink their water. Optional: add some very diluted low calorie lemonade. Available in packets. Serve in paper cups.

1. Sliced Oranges with Sliced Cucumber
2. Sliced Orange with Mashed Blueberry
3. Cut up Watermelon with Mint leaves
4. Cut up Strawberries with Squeezed Lime and Cucumber
5. Sliced Grapefruit with Rosemary
6. Mashed Blueberries with Lavender
7. Cut up Cantaloupe, Squeezed Lime and Mint leaves
8. Sliced Kiwi and Sliced Cucumber
9. Ice Tea with Crystal Light Lemonade
10. Sliced Mango and Squeezed Lime
11. Sliced Lemons and Chopped Cilantro
12. Ginger with Mint and Agave Syrup

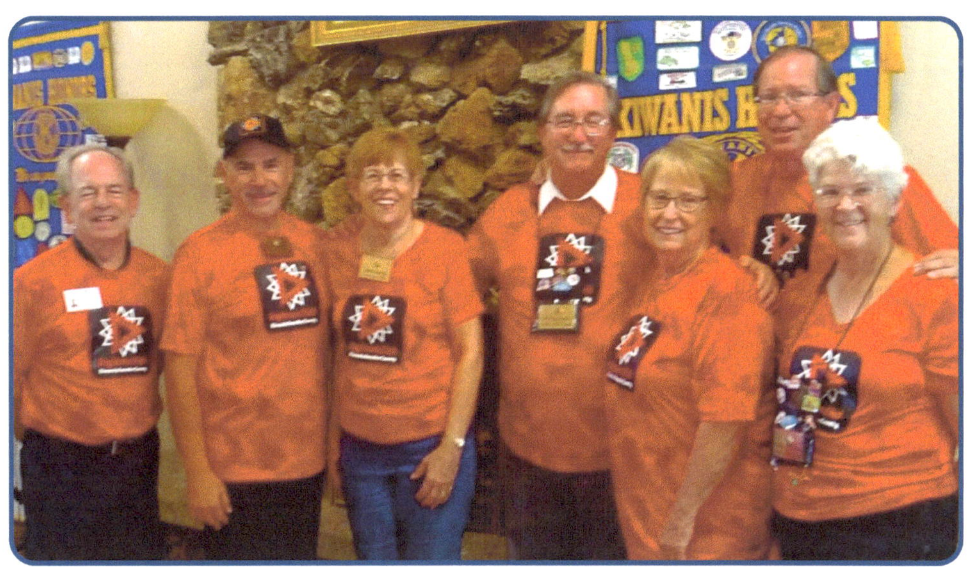

Kiwanis Righturn.Club Supporters at the Kiwanis Division 44 meeting in Sacramento. Laird Smith, Thomas Moraitis, Jane Gleason, Kevin Blasingame, Melody Anderson, Guy Blair and Debbie Blasingame.

Healthy Snacks

The kids are hungry when they arrive right after school. So provide a small apple, pear, half a banana or other fruit. You can use nuts, raisins in small paper cups, too. The snack after the run is more substantial and should involve some preparation that kids can do. Here are 12 ideas we have used. As I mentioned the local food bank was the major source, but supplements are needed sometimes. I often drop by the local grocery store and pick up a cucumber and some mint.

1. Celery sticks with peanut butter
2. Half of an orange with 1/2 cheese stick
3. Cut up seasonal fruit and cheese on a skewer
4. Cut up apples with almond butter
5. Protein peanut butter balls with raisins
6. Baked kale chips (See recipe on page 64.)
7. Whole apples, pears, oranges, other seasonal fruits.
8. Raisin, walnut mix and vanilla yogurt with graham cracker
9. Cut up watermelon, cantaloupe or honey dew
10. Small bunch of grapes
11. Pistachio and sliced apples
12. Cherries, apricots or plums

Always control portions. Serve family style in small groups. Avoid salty chips of any kind. Part of preparing snacks is to clean up afterwards. Some schools have gardens and welcome seeds, etc. for composting. Promote healthy eating and portion control when serving snacks. More on these topics in Activities.

If you have a local ice creamery in the area, it would be fun to serve some type of ice cream in a small container or small cone for a huge treat or after a difficult challenge as a reward.

> # "You don't have to eat less. You just have to eat RIGHT."

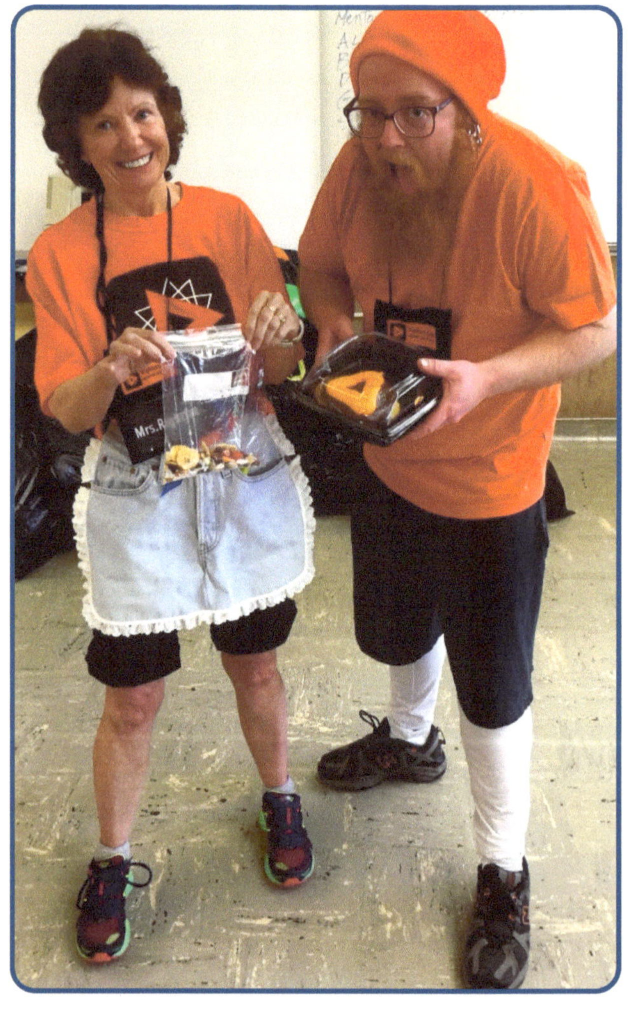

Mrs. Right Fat and Mr. Wrong Fat Skit featuring community volunteers.

RIGHT BOUNCE CARD

OPEN EGG CRATE

Kiwanis
Righturn.Club

RIGHT BOUNCE CARD

OPEN EGG CRATE

Kiwanis
Righturn.Club

RIGHT BOUNCE CARD

OPEN EGG CRATE

Kiwanis
Righturn.Club

RIGHT BOUNCE CARD

OPEN EGG CRATE

Kiwanis
Righturn.Club

RIGHT BOUNCE CARD

OPEN EGG CRATE

Kiwanis
Righturn.Club

RIGHT BOUNCE CARD

OPEN EGG CRATE

Kiwanis
Righturn.Club

Right Bounce Cards: Print six up on a letter size cover stock paper: 8.5 x11in.

Activity/Attendance Chart

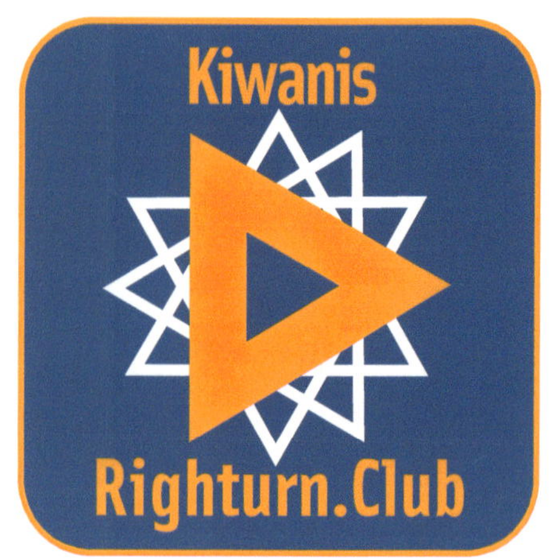

▶ Record progress and participation for each Activity and Date.
▶ Circle numbers that members attend
▶ Members will be welcomed all during the 10 week session.
▶ To be printed on card stock, thick paper.
▶ Mentors: Use a thin Marking pen to write names and circle sessions.

Name   **Grade**   **Activities/Attendance 10 Weeks** Circle Attendance

Name	Grade	1	2	3	4	5	6	7	8	9	10
1.		1 2	3 4	5 6	7 8	9 10	11 12	13 14	15 16	17 18	19 20
2.		1 2	3 4	5 6	7 8	9 10	11 12	13 14	15 16	17 18	19 20
3.		1 2	3 4	5 6	7 8	9 10	11 12	13 14	15 16	17 18	19 20
4.		1 2	3 4	5 6	7 8	9 10	11 12	13 14	15 16	17 18	19 20
5.		1 2	3 4	5 6	7 8	9 10	11 12	13 14	15 16	17 18	19 20
6.		1 2	3 4	5 6	7 8	9 10	11 12	13 14	15 16	17 18	19 20
7.		1 2	3 4	5 6	7 8	9 10	11 12	13 14	15 16	17 18	19 20
8.		1 2	3 4	5 6	7 8	9 10	11 12	13 14	15 16	17 18	19 20
9.		1 2	3 4	5 6	7 8	9 10	11 12	13 14	15 16	17 18	19 20
10.		1 2	3 4	5 6	7 8	9 10	11 12	13 14	15 16	17 18	19 20
11.		1 2	3 4	5 6	7 8	9 10	11 12	13 14	15 16	17 18	19 20
12.		1 2	3 4	5 6	7 8	9 10	11 12	13 14	15 16	17 18	19 20
13.		1 2	3 4	5 6	7 8	9 10	11 12	13 14	15 16	17 18	19 20
14.		1 2	3 4	5 6	7 8	9 10	11 12	13 14	15 16	17 18	19 20
15.		1 2	3 4	5 6	7 8	9 10	11 12	13 14	15 16	17 18	19 20
16.		1 2	3 4	5 6	7 8	9 10	11 12	13 14	15 16	17 18	19 20
17.		1 2	3 4	5 6	7 8	9 10	11 12	13 14	15 16	17 18	19 20
18.		1 2	3 4	5 6	7 8	9 10	11 12	13 14	15 16	17 18	19 20
19.		1 2	3 4	5 6	7 8	9 10	11 12	13 14	15 16	17 18	19 20
20.		1 2	3 4	5 6	7 8	9 10	11 12	13 14	15 16	17 18	19 20
21.		1 2	3 4	5 6	7 8	9 10	11 12	13 14	15 16	17 18	19 20
22.		1 2	3 4	5 6	7 8	9 10	11 12	13 14	15 16	17 18	19 20
23.		1 2	3 4	5 6	7 8	9 10	11 12	13 14	15 16	17 18	19 20
24.		1 2	3 4	5 6	7 8	9 10	11 12	13 14	15 16	17 18	19 20

School ____ **Start Date** _______________

CHAPTER 6

Game and Activity Ideas

Indoor Games

Sometimes the weather is too hot, too cold or it's raining or snowing. Although it might be fun to run in the snow, you have to run safe, and slipping is not in the program. Here are 12 indoor games and activities that are fun.

1. Juggling plastic grocery bags, followed by silk scarves. See YouTube for directions.
2. Balloon Bust: Divide group in half. Half keep them up. Half sit and bust.
3. Uptown Funk Type of Dance. Great warm up, too.
4. Indoor Folk Dancing. Country Line Dancing, Zomba or Greek…
5. Learn Cadence by writing on board. Lining up in two and each pair shouting the verses, then going to back of line.
6. Storytelling with hand gestures is a blast.
7. Circle Memory Game Pick a topic like camping gear. Say name and gear. Repeat each name/gear of each person. Next to the right does the same.
8. Mr. Right Fat and Mrs. Wrong Fat Skit, or other skits to illustrate a topic.
9. Portion Control Worksheet: Draw favorite or healthy foods on plate.
10. Balloon Follow the Leader: Place a balloon between each person, no hands. Go around the room slowly at first, then speeding up, to music. If your balloon drops in front of you, you are out. Continue until their are two winners.
11. Right Bounce Game. Using ping pong balls and egg crates. Directions: 1. Draw Card 2. Bounce Ping-Pong Balls to match pattern on card. 3. Take Card when you match it. 4. Go back to start. Whoever has the most cards wins. Play as a team or individually.
12. Using My Head: Place a pantyhose with a waffle-ball in one of the feet on your head. Swing the ball, by moving your head and strike down a standing empty water bottle.

"Good, better, best. Never let it rest. Til your good is better and your better is best." St. Jerome

Outdoor Games

Here are some variations of relay races, tag along with other games. It's fun to raise the notch in a creative way. Here are 12 outdoor games and activities that are really so much fun.

▶ 1. **Giant # Hashtag Tic Tac Toe** Cut up 4 solid color blankets into 2 ft squares for X's and O's. Make a large connecting hashtag out of 2 ft white PVC pipes with connectors. Make 4 of these. Form 4 groups with even players, half one color half the other. At the Go, Kids run up and place a color in a square. They try to get three acrosss vertically, horizontally or diagonally.

▶ 2. **Balloon Toss** Form two parallel lines of kids, give a water filled balloon to each kid on one side. Be one step apart. Throw ballons to teammate. Take one step back. Throw balloons. Repeat until all but one balloon is busted

Shopping List

▶ 1. 32 Kiwanis Righturn.Club shirts for Kids, 16 Shirts for adults, total of 48

▶ 2. Name Badges for 48.

▶ 3. Color and Black Markers for activities

▶ 4. Orange Balloons for indoor play 144.

▶ 5. Orange Cones for games, 12.

▶ 6. Scarves for juggling, 72 3 colors.

▶ 7. Portable Speaker for music.

▶ 8. Knifes, peelers, orange, plates, cups, for food preparation.

▶ 9. Gallon Jugs for water beverage.

▶ 10. Tape measure, scale, stopwatch.

▶ 11. Paper: Card stock and copier.

▶ 12. White PVC Pipe and fittings for giant Ticktacktoe Game and Solid Color Blankets, cut into squares.

▶ 13. Hats, Plastic Frames for Certificates

▶ 14. Backing for Refrigerator Magnets.

▶ 15. Small gifts like Play Dough as incentives.

▶ 16. Crazy Sunglasses, 32 pair

▶ 17. Golf Ball, Baseball, deck of cards, AA Battery, Salad Plate, Light Bulb for Portion Control

▶ 18. Ping Pong Balls, Egg Crates, Cards

▶ 19. Yoga Workout Video for Children

▶ 20. Righturn.Club Banner

▶ 21. Righturn.Club Table Cloth

▶ 22. Orange Balls, various sizes

▶ 23. Index Cards 120 quantity

"Just Do It." Nike

▶ 3. **Clockwork Ball Toss** If you have 24 kids, form 2 circles, a smaller 8 ft diameter and a 20 ft diameter. Place orange cones at the time slots. 12 o'clock on top, 6 o'clock on the bottom, etc. Shout a time. Throw a large ball for the hour hand, a smaller ball for the minute hand. Between numbers, kids run around until you say stop. They change numbers each time. Fun. Lots of laughs!

▶ 4. **Orange Ball Relay** Form 4 even teams. Have a basket of different size balls, from giant 24 in plastic beach balls to ping pong balls. Place cones 15 yds away from each team. Team mates run with ball in different ways from under neck, between two people to kicking ball. Make it fun and creative. Put your own twist to this relay race.

▶ 5. **Cadence Jog** Hand out cadence cards. Kids run in pairs, in short steps to words of cadence for one mile, half mile out, half mile back. Shouting the verses. They take turns shouting the two verses, then going to the back of the pack as they jog slowly.

▶ 6. **Aerobic Dance 12 Steps** To upbeat music, kids will follow the leader.
Repeat steps, making sure each kid is doing the moves.

1. **Bounce and Twist** Bounce up and down. Feet together. Twist upper body opposite to lower body.
2. **Downhill Skier** Jump side to side, both feet together, lift alternate arms to the side.
3. **Elbow to Knee** Alternate lifting the knees, touching each with the opposite elbow.
4. **Hopscotch** hands on waist, hop in place, alternating feet, bending the lifted knee to the back
   with each hop.
5. **Jumping Jacks** Stand straight with arms at side. Jump up, landing with feet apart, and arms
   extended overhead. Return to starting position.
6. **Knee Slap** Alternate lifting the knees, touching each with both hands at the same time.
7. **Leg Kicks** Alternating between legs, hop on one foot while kicking the other out in front.
8. **Lunge** Stand, feet together. Jump to the right, landing on right foot, forward, left foot back.
   Return to start jump to left, on left foot forward, right foot back. Extend arms overhead
   with each lunge.
9. **Pedalium Swing** legs side to side, hopping on one four at a time.
10. **March in Place** Alternate lifting the knees, swinging the arms in opposition.
11. **Stride Jump** Stand with one foot in front of the other. Jump up and switch feet, landing with
    the other foot in front.
12. **Super Ball** Bounce up and down on the balls of the feet. Let the heels touch the floor before
    bouncing back up again.
Dancing is fun. You could also add some dance moves here and there. Add a light, laser show!

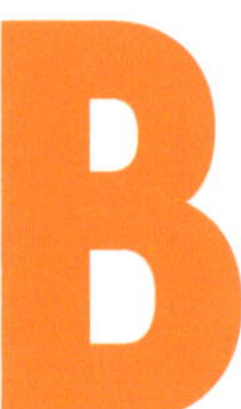

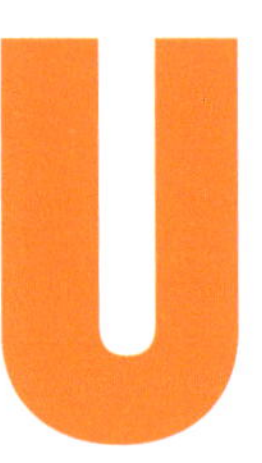

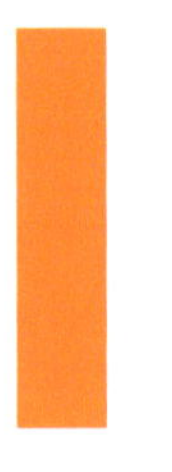

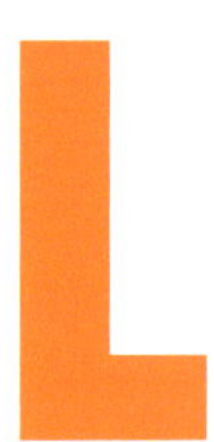

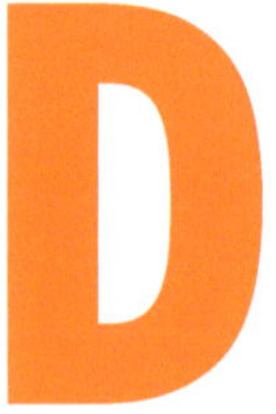

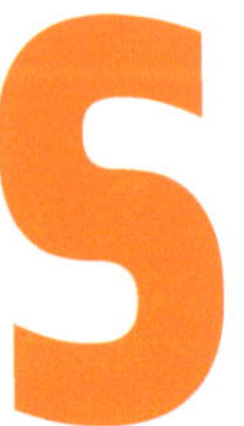

1. Name a dairy food high in protein.

2. Name a breakfast food high in protein.

3. Name a beverage high in protein.

4. Name a meat high in protein.

5. Name a seafood high in protein.

6. Name a poultry food high in protein.

Note: Not sure what the answers are? Go online and search.

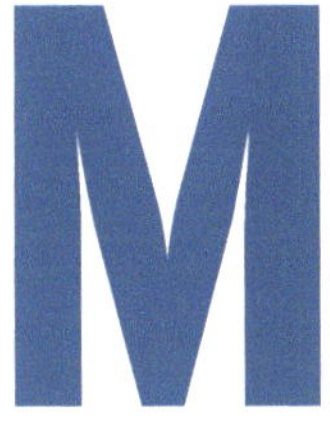

7. Name a canned food high in protein.

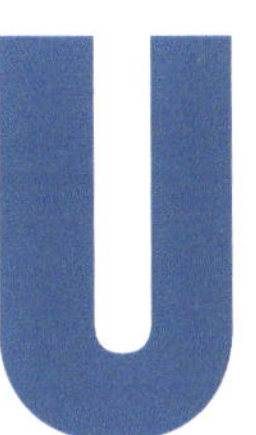

8. Name a deli food high in protein.

9. Name a snack high in protein.

10. Name a nut product high in protein.

11. Name a vegetable high in protein.

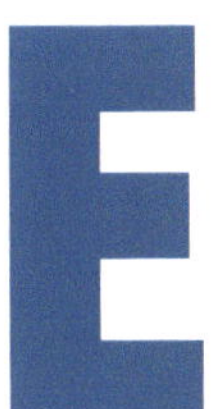

12. Name your all-time favorite high protein food.

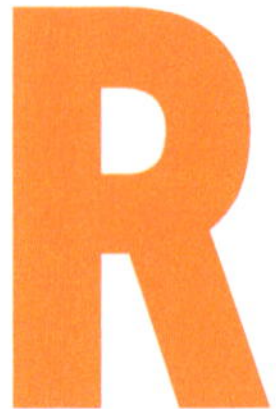

1. Name something to eat using halfsies.

2. Name something to eat that is a right fat or good fat.

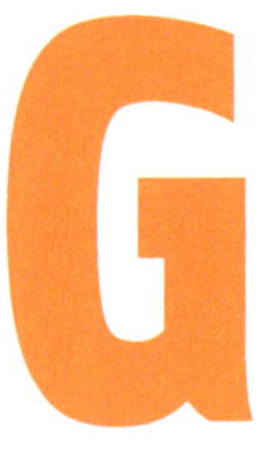

3. Name something to eat that is a wrong fat or bad fat.

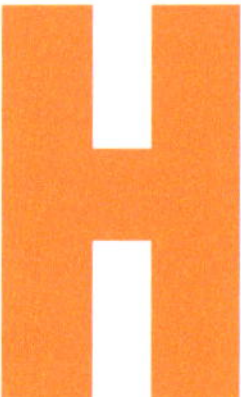

4. What is the right portion for the size of cheese?

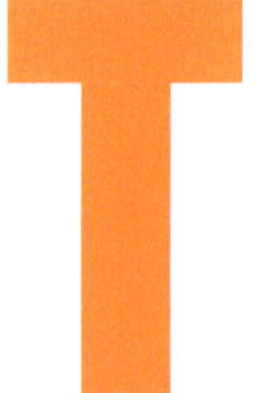

5. What is the right portion for the size of meat?

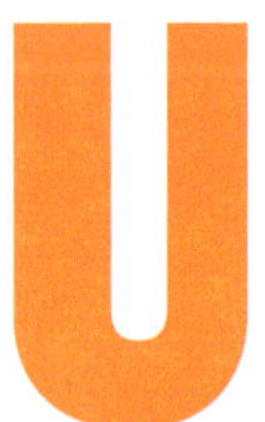

6. What is the right portion for the size for veggies?

Note: Not sure what the answers are? Go online and search.

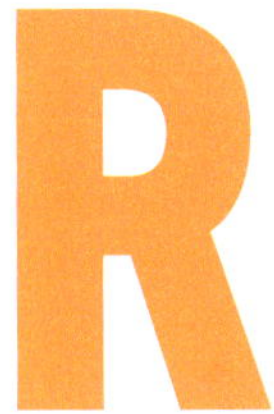

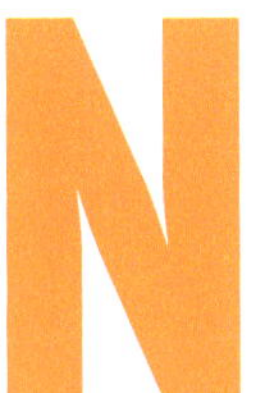

7. What should you wear to Righturn.Club each time?

8. Why should you run with a friend?

9. Why should you eat protein everyday?

10. Why should you avoid drinking soda?

11. What have you learned that changed the way you eat?

12. What is your favorite game or activity you learned?

Help Kids Get Fit and Choose Healthy!

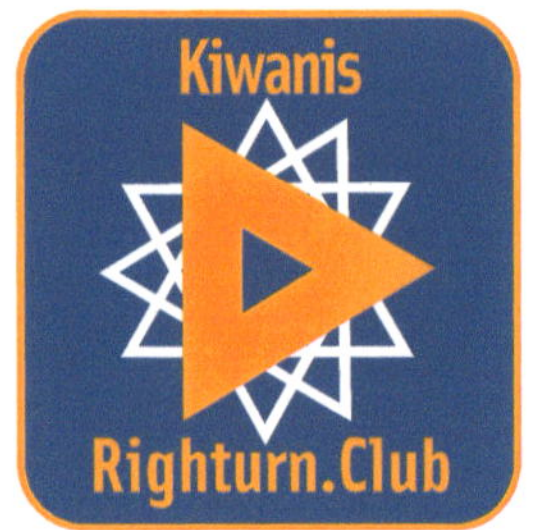

School:________________

Time:________________

Dates:________________

Call for Mentors, Helpers and Volunteers

The Need To Make A Right Turn

▶ Ready to give back to your community? Have some free time for 10 weeks, meeting twice a week for 1 hour?

▶ We are the choices we make. Help kids be more active and make better choices with your help as a mentor.

▶ It's time to do what's right. Right now.

How to Volunteer in Righturn.Club

▶ Fill out the Mentor Application Form

▶ Don't delay. You will be required to do a fingerprint scan, a TB test and Mentor Training before meeting the kids.

▶ Other volunteers are needed. Contact ________________ at ________________ for details.

▶ All volunteers are welcome.

▶ Volunteer TODAY!

Righturn.Club Is...

▶ ...a fitness program focused on kids who want to get fit and make better food choices with the help of a Mentor.

Contact Info:________________

Volunteer Flyer: Print three up on a legal size paper: 8.5 x14in.

9. **Follow the Leader** Select someone to lead. Form a snake. Have a loud drum. Every minute or so make a loud beat, leader goes to back of line, new leader takes over. Hop (both feet or one foot), skip, jump, roll, sideways, backwards, side by side steps, Hands on head, They just have to keep moving. You can also use music, and stop the music every minute or so to change leaders.

10. **Timed One Mile Run** At a track, place orange cones as a start/lap marker. Kids run 4 laps around the track. Mentors shout time as they pass by. This is recorded on there My Statistics Form. When fast kids finish, they encourage the other to go.

11. **4,3 2 1, Go!** Place 12 cones in a large circle like a clock. The size of the circle will vary, but use a grass area, a baseball field is ideal. The Members run one min. then walk one min. Next run 2 min., walk 2 min. Next run 3 min., walk 3 min. Finally run 4 min., walk 4 min.

12. **Alphabet Tag** On a grassy field divide kids into two even groups. Line up on opposite sides of a space the size of a basketball court. Assign one member to be the leader, who will shout out a letter at the sideline. Each kid with that last name runs acrosss the field. Assign 3 members to be inside the field in the middle. They will try to tag the runner. If they succeed, they can join the other side. If they get tagged they join the taggers in the middle of the field. Kids on the perimeters shout out their letter for the first name so they can run.

Mentoring Members of Righturn.Club

When we work with and mentor Righturn.Club members during projects and activities, their care and welfare are being entrusted to us. The school district and Kiwanis International have youth protection guidelines that we follow for everyone who has any contact with kids. "Kiwanians in particular have good reason to act with the highest standards. If we want to be the premier provider of youth service clubs and programs, we need to hold ourselves and our fellow members to the highest standards of conduct and awareness."

Who wants to be a Mentor?

▶ A high school student who needs to earn public service hours and likes to run.

▶ A parent who is excited that their child is actively involved in the club and has time to volunteer.

▶ A teacher, who loves to run and wants to see her kids learn about eating healthy and becoming more active in a setting outside of the classroom.

▶ A Kiwanian or community member who wants to be involved with a hands on program to help kids directly in their hometown.

▶ An employee of an organization that promotes community philanthropy.

▶ A child who has completed the program and wants to mentor other friends.

How to Volunteer as a Mentor

▶ Fill out the Mentor Application Form. Have the time in your schedule.

▶ Don't delay. You will be required to fill out a school form for volunteers, complete a fingerprint scan and a TB test

▶ All volunteers are welcome, regardless of size, shape or degree of fitness.

Kiwanis International Youth Protection Guidelines

The following guidelines are taken from the Kiwanis International Web Site. The content is edited for Mentors serving at Elementary Schools. Rules about overnight stays and transportation were not included.

▶ Chaperone

A chaperone is defined as a Kiwanis member, faculty member, parent, legal guardian, or person who is in the place of a parent, 21 years of age or older, who has been approved by the school or agency and registered with the school or agency to accompany the youth members at the specific event.

▶ Criminal History Background Checks

Kiwanis Clubs are required to have a clear criminal history background check conducted and verified by Kiwanis International of any member serving as a Kiwanis advisor to any Service Leadership Program club and Kiwanis Righturn.Club. Kiwanis International's criteria shall be followed to determine whether the background check is considered 'clear.' Background checks shall be valid for no more than two years. Kiwanis Clubs are strongly encouraged to ensure confidential background checks for all adults who will work directly with youth outside of the school and/or who may not have undergone a background check. The criminal history background check should conform to applicable local and state/provincial laws and requirements. Kiwanis International requires clear criminal history background checks conducted by its provider for all adults working with youth at all Kiwanis International-sponsored events , including Kiwanis Righturn.Club.

▶ Transportation

When transporting youth, the best practice is having three people in the car at all times with documented approval from the parent or guardian for the transportation arrangements. When both of these conditions cannot be met, one of them should be. All transportation decisions should be made in accordance with local laws and school policies.

▶ Use of Alcoholic Beverages, Tobacco, Marijuana, and Other Substances

While attending any Kiwanis event that is produced primarily by or for the benefit of youth, adults are expected to refrain from using or being under the influence of alcoholic beverages, tobacco, and/or marijuana products, even if prescribed for medicinal use. In addition, the use and/or possession of illegal drugs or the improper/illegal use of legal drugs is prohibited.

▶ Medications

The possession of prescription and nonprescription (over-the-counter) medications by youth at a Kiwanis event should be permitted only with the written permission of the parent/guardian.

▶ Reporting

If a Kiwanian observes troubling behavior involving a youth at a Kiwanis event or becomes aware of a situation on that is illegal or potentially unsafe for a young person at a Kiwanis event, he or she must immediately contact the appropriate personnel at the event and provide notification to law enforcement personnel as appropriate. If the Kiwanian becomes aware of the troubling behavior after the event, he/she must contact leaders of the event and provide notification to law enforcement personnel as appropriate. All local, state, provincial and federal laws regarding reporting must be followed.

▶ Personal Information

All documents, including registration forms, medical information forms, permission-to-treat forms, etc. should be treated as confidential. Processes that protect this information must be created, including minimizing the number of people who have access to any such documents. The documents shall be maintained for a minimum of three years or longer as may be required by applicable state/provincial laws and regulations.

▶ Behavioral or Health Issues

Kiwanians are often seen by a young person as an adult to trust with personal and/or sensitive information. Kiwanians should refrain from counseling youth and should instead find, or assist the young person in finding, appropriate expert assistance.

▶ Youth and Social Media

For any social networking site that involves requesting a connection (such as inviting someone to be a friend on Facework), adults should never initiate such connections with youth.

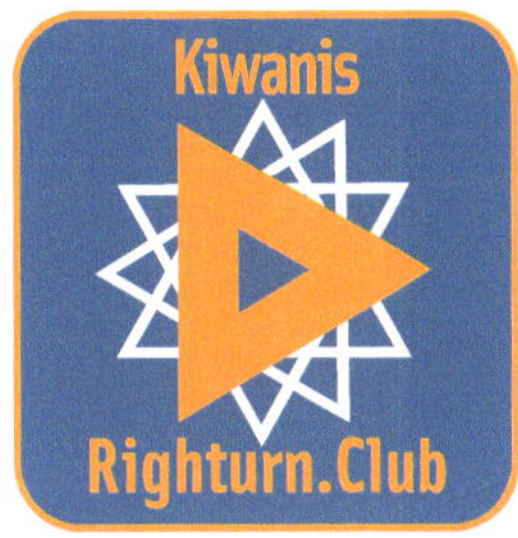

Join Righturn.Club— Meets After School

School:________________
Time:________________
Dates:________________

Run, Play Games and Hang Out with Friends

What is it?

An afterschool running club.

Why?

To eat healthier and be more active and have fun!

What do you do?

Meet, dance, play, run and get free snacks.

What time?

Starts after shool, twice a week and goes for 2 hrs.

How do I join?

Sign up, get your parent permission

Contact Info:________________________________

Student Flyer: Print three up on a legal size paper: 8.5 x14 in.

Help Your Child Get Fit and Choose Healthy!

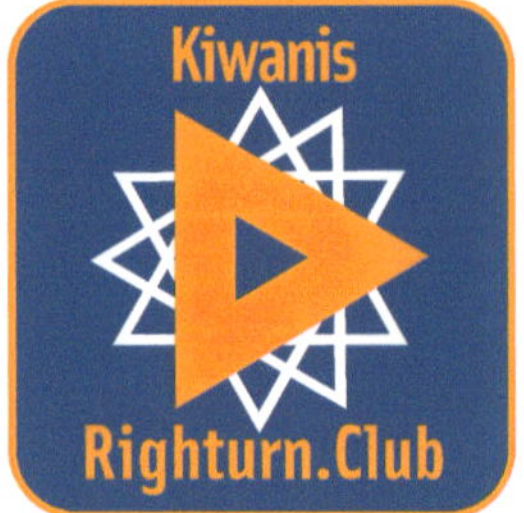

School:_________________

Time:_________________

Dates:_________________

Enroll Your Child Today

The Need To Make A Right Turn

▶ Is your child over eating? Are they less active than you were, when you were their age?

▶ We are the choices we make. Your child may need our help in order to make better choices.

▶ It's time to do what's right. Right now.

How to Enroll Your Child in Righturn.Club

▶ Pick up Student Information Form at Front Office of School

▶ Volunteer as a helper or Mentor if you are available.

▶ Make some better choices when it comes to meal preparation and family activities. Eat smaller portions and take walks together.

Righturn.Club Is...

▶ ...A fitness program focused on kids who want to get fit and make better food choices with the help of a Mentor.

▶ ...3-5 kids meet with Mentors (teens and adults from the community) after school, twice a week for 10 weeks.

Contact Info:_________________

Parents Flyer: Print three up on a legal size paper: 8.5 x14in.

If a youth requests such a connection from a Kiwanian, he/she should use their best judgment in responding. Adults should treat their interaction with youth on social networking sites as though the interaction were occurring in public, in front of other adults and young people. In other words, if it would not be appropriate to say something to a young person in public, it should not be said as a comment on a social networking site either. Kiwanians should refrain from interactions that can be seen as excessive (such as constantly "liking" or commenting on a person's posts on FaceBook). Prior to posting any media online, such as photographs, obtain permission from any and all individuals (or parents for minors) who appear in those media; it could be illegal to do otherwise.

▶ **Conflicts with Other Rules**

Whenever these guidelines conflict with local school policies or rules, or local state/provincial, or national laws or regulations, the highest applicable standards for conduct shall prevail.

For further information please go to http://www.kiwanis.org/kiwanisone/lead/risk-management/youth-protection-guidelines

Artwork for Righturn.Club

T-Shirt Artwork: Print 2-Color, Pantone 295 and White on a Bright Orange Shirt.

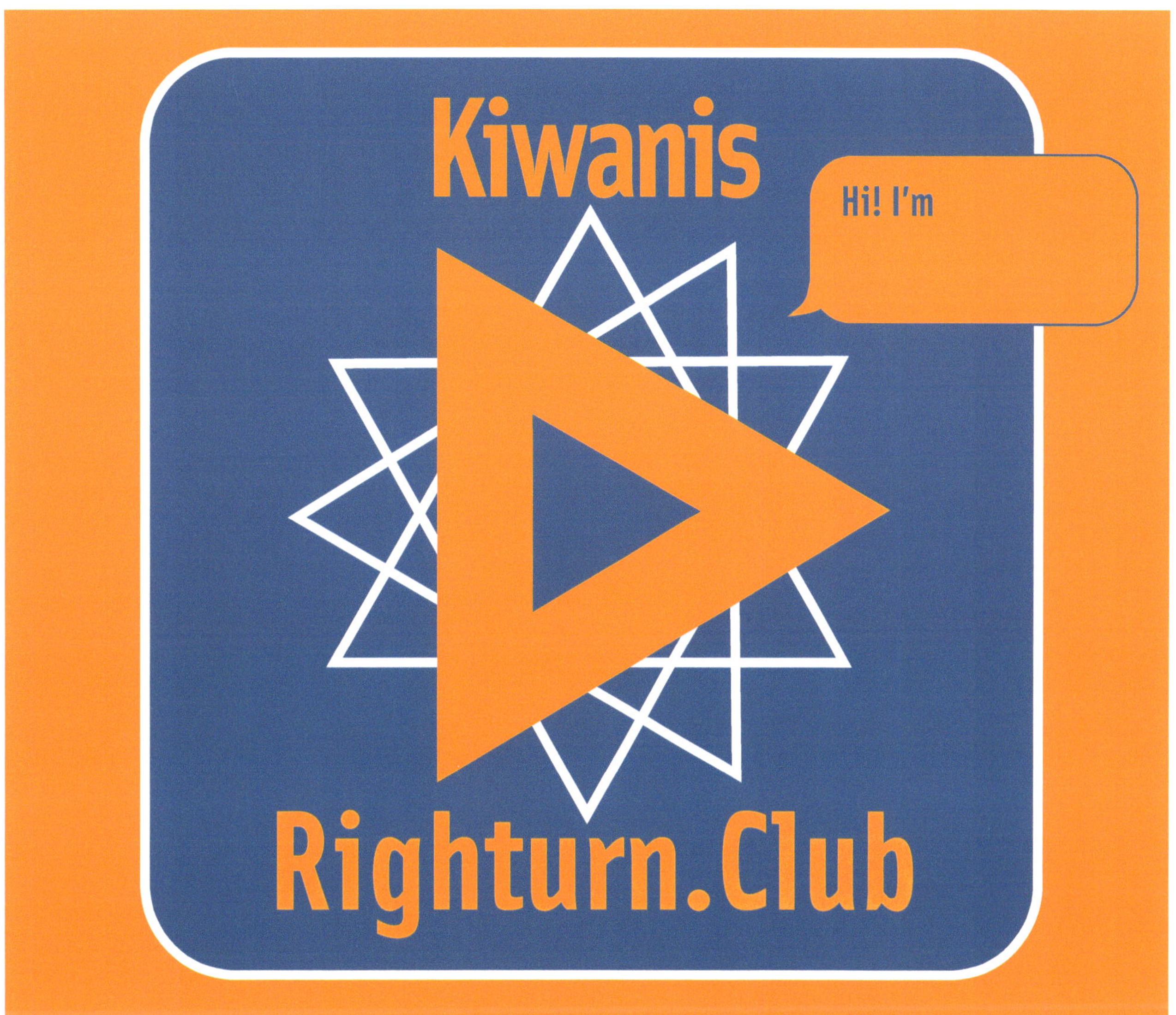

"If you fall behind, run faster. Never give up, never surrender, and RISE UP against the odds." Jesse Jackson

RISE UP has been my inspirational theme during this life changing process.

AWARD OF EXCELLENCE

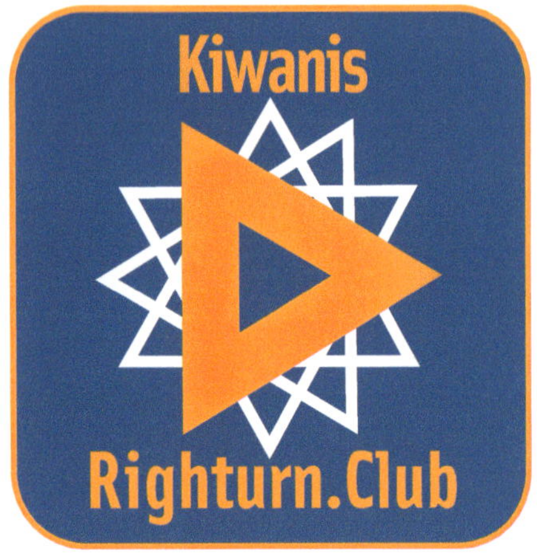

Presented To

____

Righturn.Club Member

____

School

__________________________   __________________________

Righturn.Club Mentor   Righturn.Club Mentor

RIGHTURN.CLUB IS...

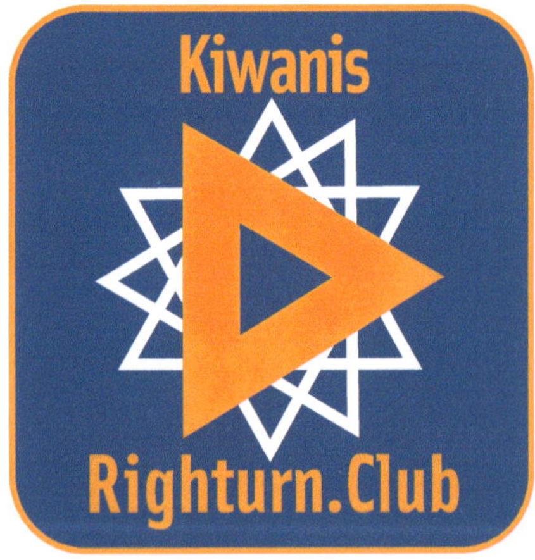

____

Righturn.Club Member

____

Grade, Date

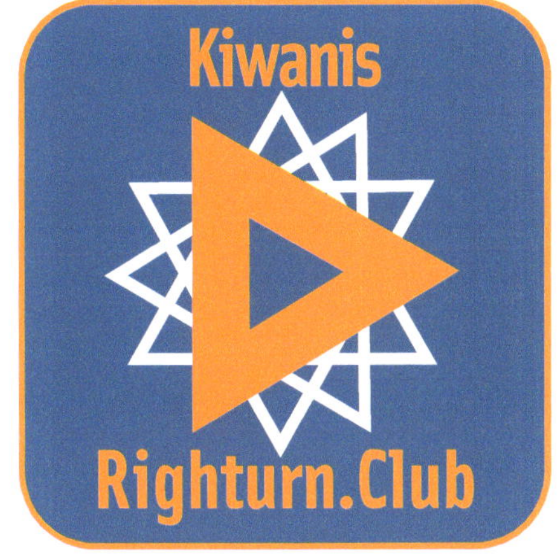

FIVE A DAY

Name ________________________________

Righturn.Club Five A Day Worksheet

Record in the space below your 5 days of High 5. List the names of the fruit and veggies you ate. Before you go to bed each night, fill this out. If you ate more than 5, list these, too.

Yesterday_____	Today________	________day	________day	________day
1._______	1._______	1._______	1._______	1._______
2._______	2._______	2._______	2._______	2._______
3._______	3._______	3._______	3._______	3._______
4._______	4._______	4._______	4._______	4._______
5._______	5._______	5._______	5._______	5._______
+._______	+._______	+._______	+._______	+._______
+._______	+._______	+._______	+._______	+._______
+._______	+._______	+._______	+._______	+._______
+._______	+._______	+._______	+._______	+._______
+._______	+._______	+._______	+._______	+._______
+._______	+._______	+._______	+._______	+._______

Fruits	Cranberries	Nectarines	Raspberries	Beets	Cilantro	Green Onions	Sprouts
Apples	Dates	Oranges	Strawberries	Broccoli	Collard	Kale	String
Apricots	Figs	Papaya	Watermelon	Brussel	Greens	Lettuce	Beans
Bananas	Grapefruit	Peaches	**Vegetables**	Sprouts	Corn	Mushrooms	Squash
Blackberries	Grapes	Pineapple	Artichoke	Cabbage	Cucumbers	Onions	Sweet
Blueberries	Kiwi	Plums	Arugula	Carrots	Eggplant	Peppers, Bell	Potatoes
Cantaloupe	Lemons	Prunes	Asparagus	Cauliflower	Fennel	Potatoes	Swiss Chard
Cherries	Limes	Pomegranate	Avocado	Celery	Garlic	Peas	Tomatoes
Coconut	Melon	Raisins	Basil	Chives	Ginger	Spinach	Zucchini

"Five A Day gives you energy to play."

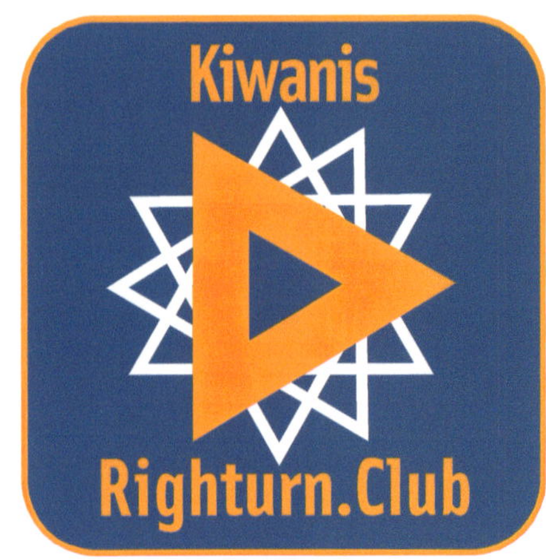

Fitness and Nutrition Assessment

Place your answer letter by the number.

Name ______________________________   What did you eat yesterday?   Dinner ______________________________

Grade __________ Age __________   Breakfast ______________________   ______________________________

Time:______________________________   ______________________________   ______________________________

Hight __________ Weight __________   Lunch ______________________   Snacks ______________________________

School ______________________________   ______________________________   ______________________________

Answers   **Complete each sentence with your best answer for today.**

1. _____   1. I drink water   A. never B. 1-2 times C. 3-4 times D. 5-6 or more times a day.

2. _____   2. I go outside and play A. never B. 1-2 times C. 3-4 times D. 5-6 or more times a day.

3. _____   3. I eat candy, soda pop A. never B. 1-2 times C. 3-4 times D. 5-6 or more times a day.

4. _____   4. I eat cookies, cake A. never B. 1-2 times C. 3-4 times D. 5-6 or more times a day.

5. _____   5. I eat fresh fruit A. never B. 1-2 times C. 3-4 times D. 5-6 or more times a day.

6. _____   6. I eat vegetables A. never B. 1-2 times C. 3-4 times D. 5-6 or more times a day.

7. _____   7. I add sugar to food A. never B. 1-2 times C. 3-4 times D. 5-6 or more times a day.

8. _____   8. I like a second helping   A. never B. 1-2 times C. 3-4 times D. 5-6 or more times a day.

9. _____   9. I play video games A. never B. 1-2 times C. 3-4 times D. 5-6 or more times a day.

10. _____   10. I am on my phone   A. never B. 1-2 times C. 3-4 times D. 5-6 or more times a day.

11. _____   11. I run or hike outside A. never B. 1-2 times C. 3-4 times D. 5-6 or more times a day.

12. _____   12. I often share half my food A. never B. 1-2 times C. 3-4 times D. 5-6 times a day.

13. _____   13. I like to exercise with a friend A. never B. 1-2 times C. 3-4 times D. 5-6 times a day.

14. _____   14. I eat more than I should A. never B. 1-2 times C. 3-4 times D. 5-6 times a day.

15. _____   15. I eat healthy snacks A. never B. 1-2 times C. 3-4 times D. 5-6 times a day.

16. _____   16. I eat unhealthy snacks A. never B. 1-2 times C. 3-4 times D. 5-6 times a day.

17. _____   17. I drink diet soda A. never B. 1-2 times C. 3-4 times D. 5-6 times a day.

18. _____   18. I ride my bike A. never B. 1-2 times C. 3-4 times D. 5-6 times a day.

19. _____   19. I share some foods with others A. never B. 1-2 times C. 3-4 times D. 5-6 times a day.

20. _____   20. I plan on using what I learn here A. never B. 1-2 times C. 3-4 times D. 5-6 times a day.

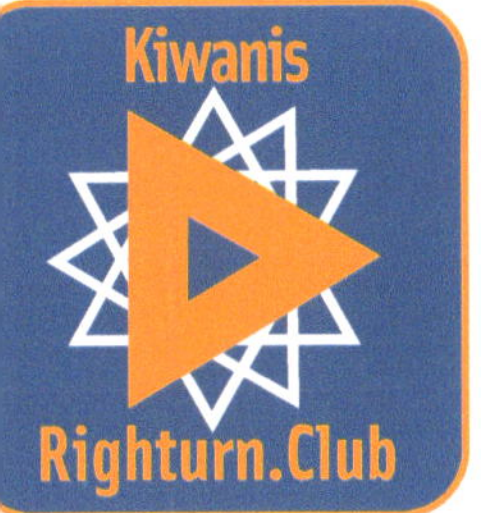

MY TURN!
Activity ____
Use back if needed.

Name ________________________________

Comment ________________________________

____

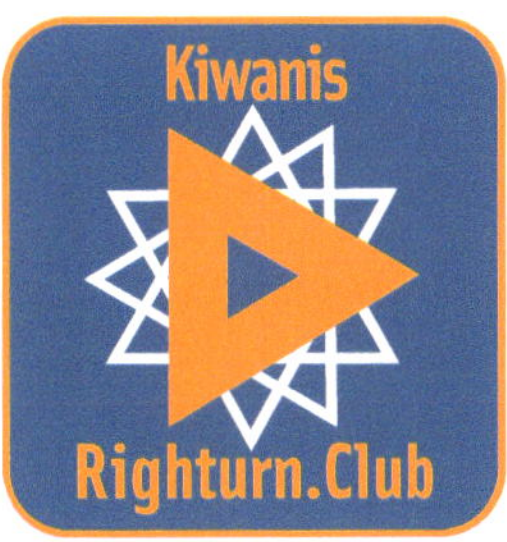

MY TURN!
Activity ____
Use back if needed.

Name ________________________________

Comment ________________________________

____

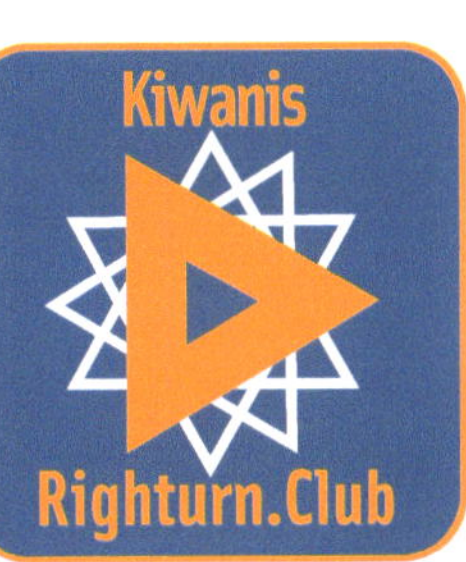

MY TURN!
Activity ____
Use back if needed.

Name ________________________________

Comment ________________________________

____

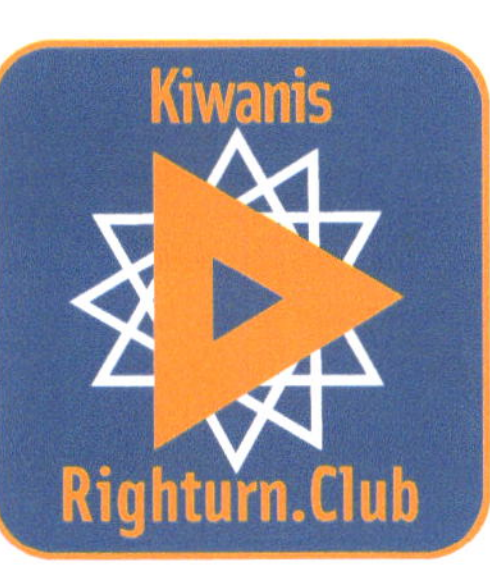

MY TURN!
Activity ____
Use back if needed.

Name ________________________________

Comment ________________________________

____

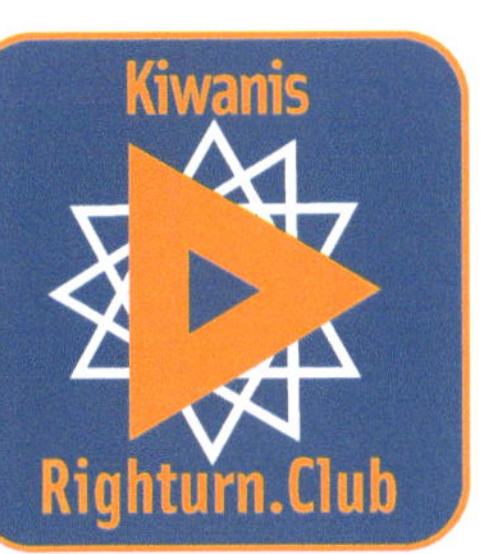

MY TURN!
Activity ____
Use back if needed.

Name ________________________________

Comment ________________________________

____

MY TURN!
Activity ____
Use back if needed.

Name ________________________________

Comment ________________________________

____

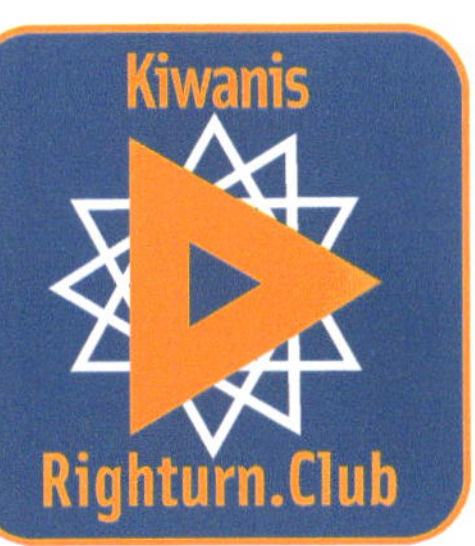

MY TURN!
Activity ____
Use back if needed.

Name ________________________________

Comment ________________________________

____

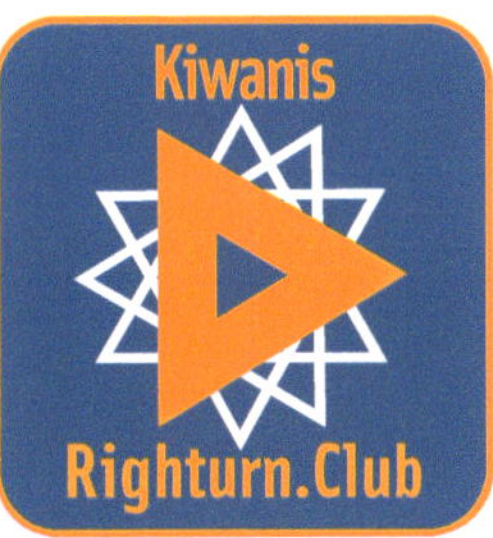

MY TURN!
Activity ____
Use back if needed.

Name ________________________________

Comment ________________________________

____

Kiwanis
Righturn.Club

PORTION PATROL
The Right Portions

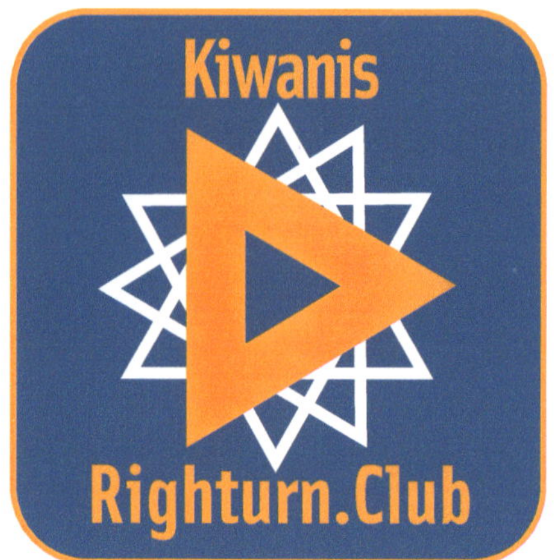

Name ______________________________

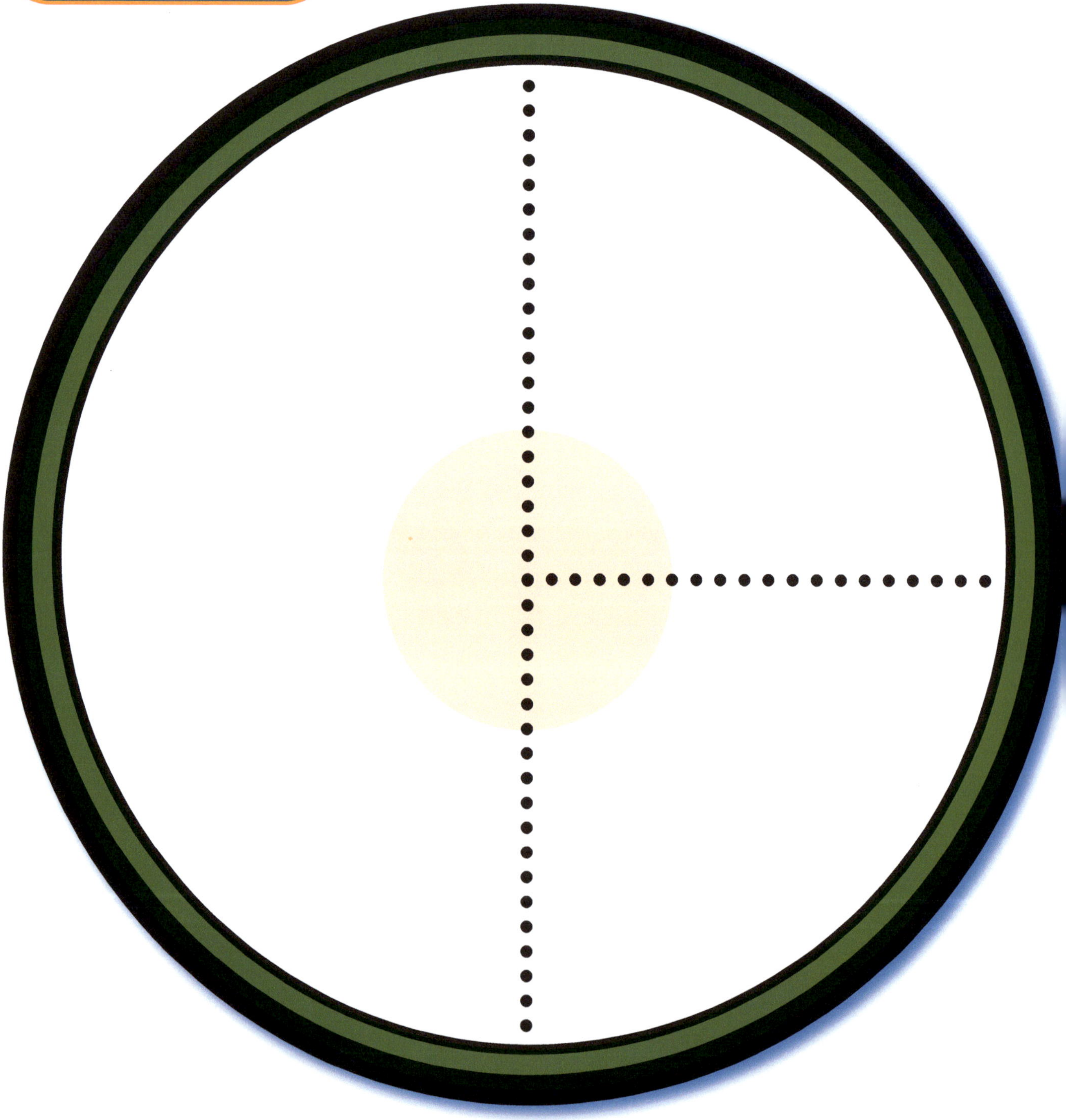

Carrots, Broccoli
Chips, Grapes, Juice

____

____

One Half Cheese Stick
4 Cheese Cubes

____

____

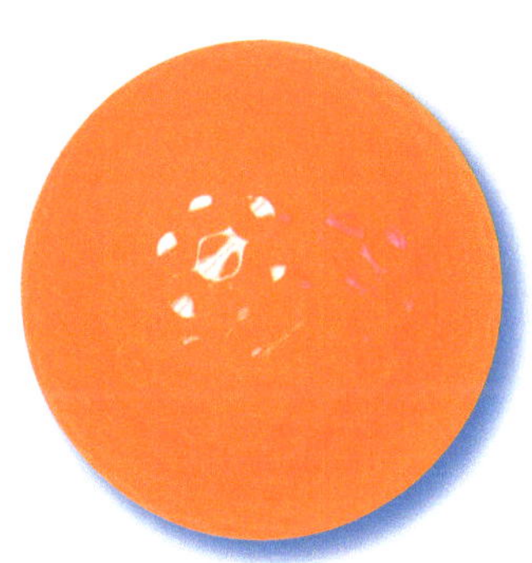

Peanut Butter, Nuts
Dried Fruit

____

____

Chicken, Burger
 Salmon

____

____

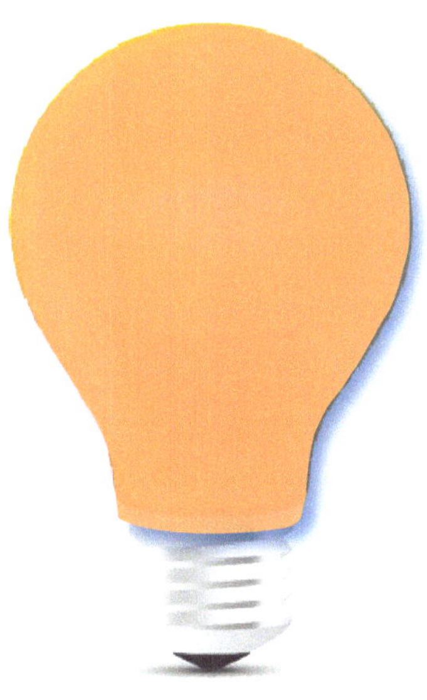

Rice, Pasta
One Slice Bread

____

____

Membership and Cadence Cards: Print six up on a letter size cover stock paper: 8.5 x11in.

MEMBERSHIP & ACTIVITY CARD

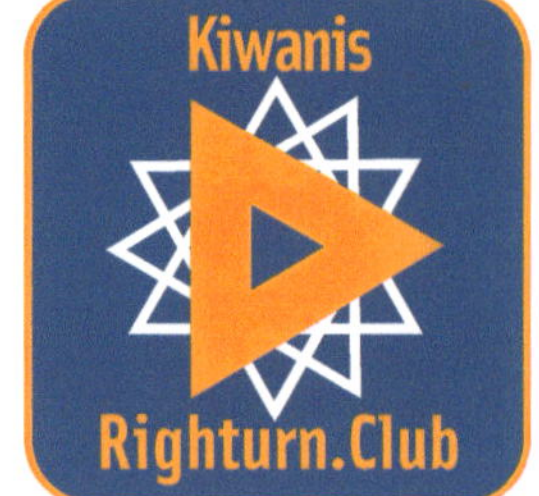

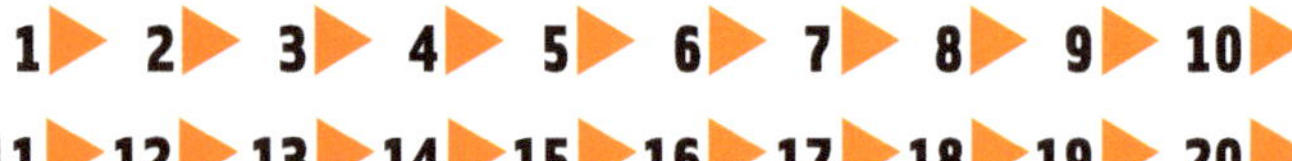

Righturn.Club Member

Elementary School

1 ▶ 2 ▶ 3 ▶ 4 ▶ 5 ▶ 6 ▶ 7 ▶ 8 ▶ 9 ▶ 10 ▶
11 ▶ 12 ▶ 13 ▶ 14 ▶ 15 ▶ 16 ▶ 17 ▶ 18 ▶ 19 ▶ 20 ▶

RIGHTURN CADENCE CARD

▶ Righturn Club you can't go wrong! *Repeat all phrases*

▶ Mentor led and going strong! ▶ All Right!

▶ Be Right! ▶ Do Right!

▶ Go Right! ▶ So Right!

▶ Join the club and have a ball!

▶ Righturn.Club is fun for all!

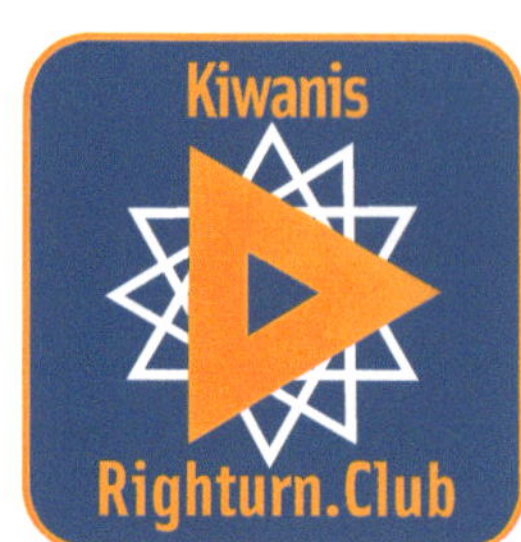

MEMBERSHIP & ACTIVITY CARD

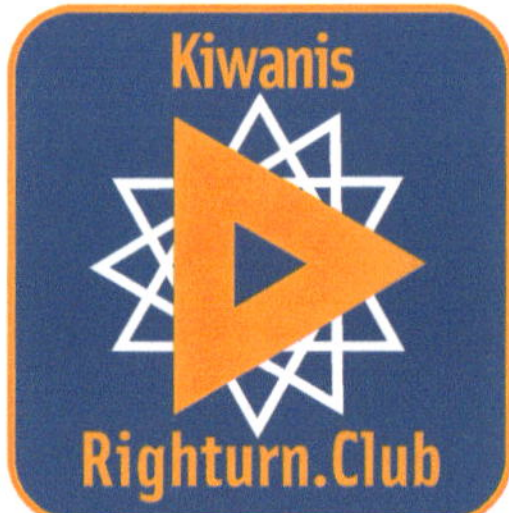

Righturn.Club Member

Elementary School

1 ▶ 2 ▶ 3 ▶ 4 ▶ 5 ▶ 6 ▶ 7 ▶ 8 ▶ 9 ▶ 10 ▶
11 ▶ 12 ▶ 13 ▶ 14 ▶ 15 ▶ 16 ▶ 17 ▶ 18 ▶ 19 ▶ 20 ▶

RIGHTURN CADENCE CARD

▶ Righturn Club you can't go wrong! *Repeat all phrases*

▶ Mentor led and going strong! ▶ All Right!

▶ Be Right! ▶ Do Right!

▶ Go Right! ▶ So Right!

▶ Join the club and have a ball!

▶ Righturn.Club is fun for all!

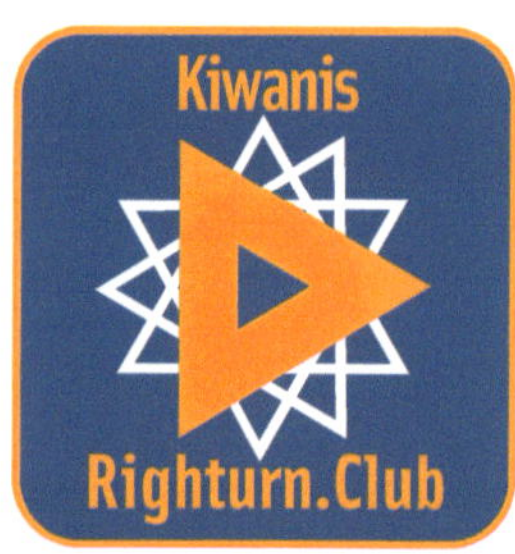

MEMBERSHIP & ACTIVITY CARD

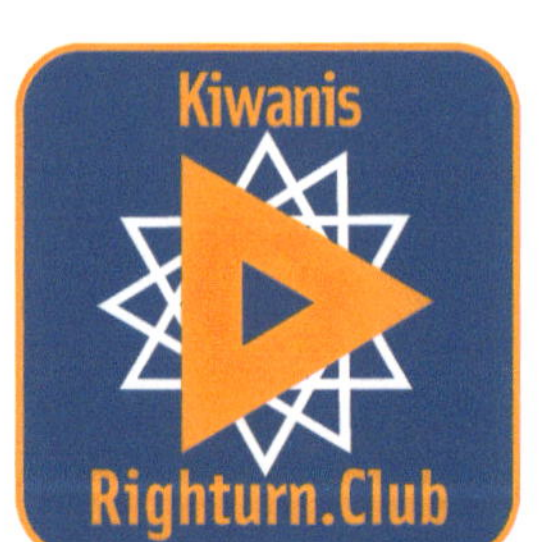

Righturn.Club Member

Elementary School

1 ▶ 2 ▶ 3 ▶ 4 ▶ 5 ▶ 6 ▶ 7 ▶ 8 ▶ 9 ▶ 10 ▶
11 ▶ 12 ▶ 13 ▶ 14 ▶ 15 ▶ 16 ▶ 17 ▶ 18 ▶ 19 ▶ 20 ▶

RIGHTURN CADENCE CARD

▶ Righturn Club you can't go wrong! *Repeat all phrases*

▶ Mentor led and going strong! ▶ All Right!

▶ Be Right! ▶ Do Right!

▶ Go Right! ▶ So Right!

▶ Join the club and have a ball!

▶ Righturn.Club is fun for all!

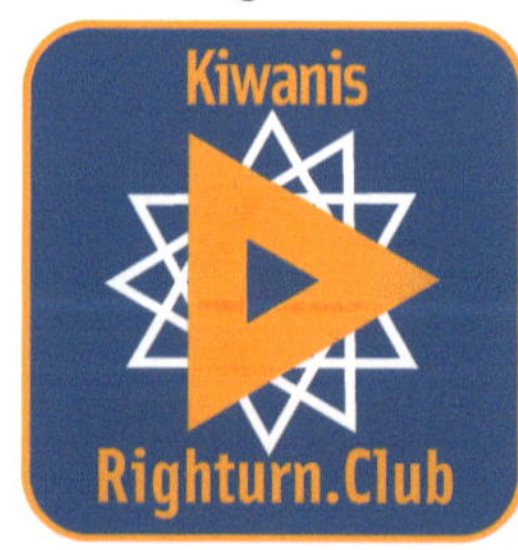

Magnets: Print on letter size plastic paper, trim, and back with flat magnets: 8.5 x11in.

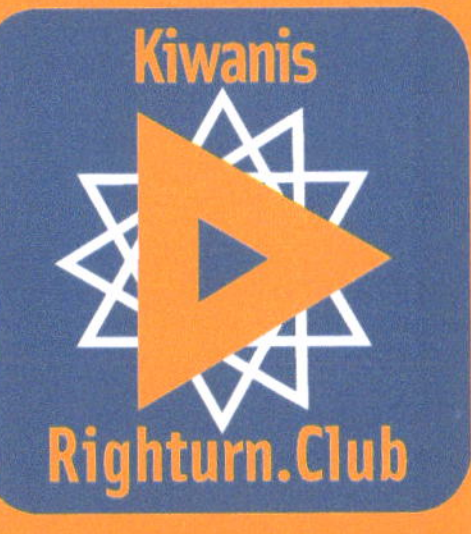

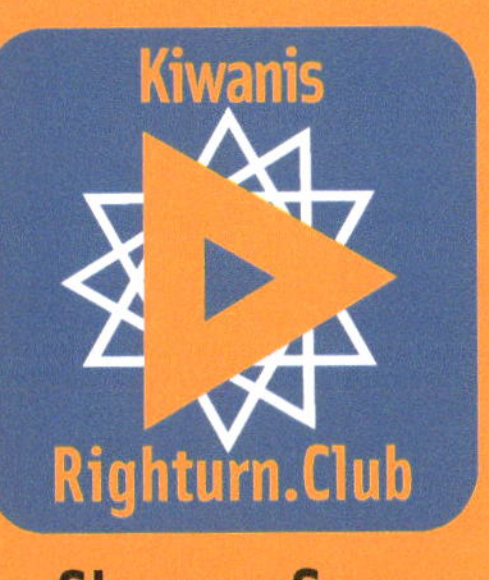

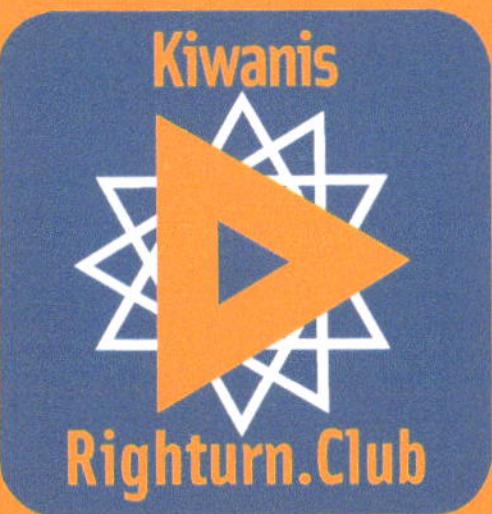

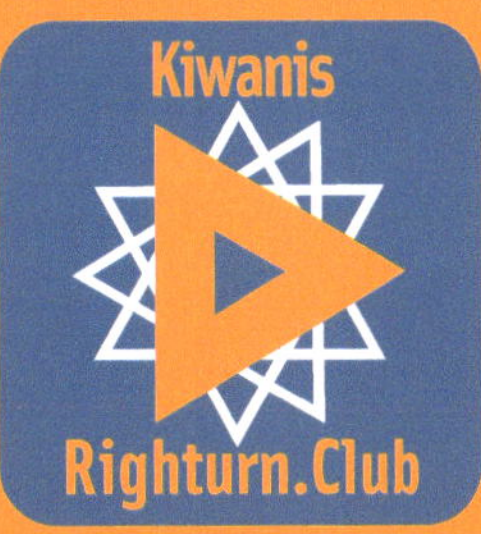

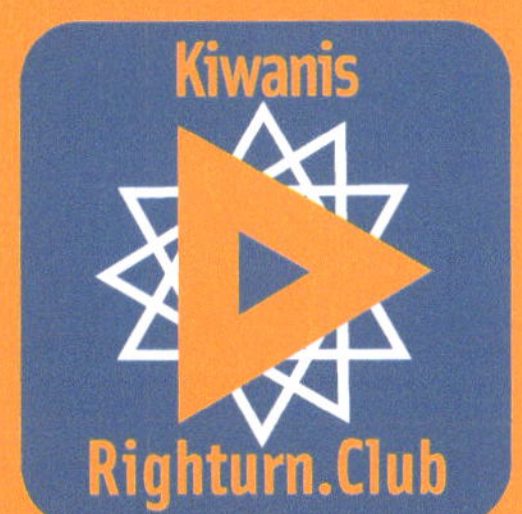

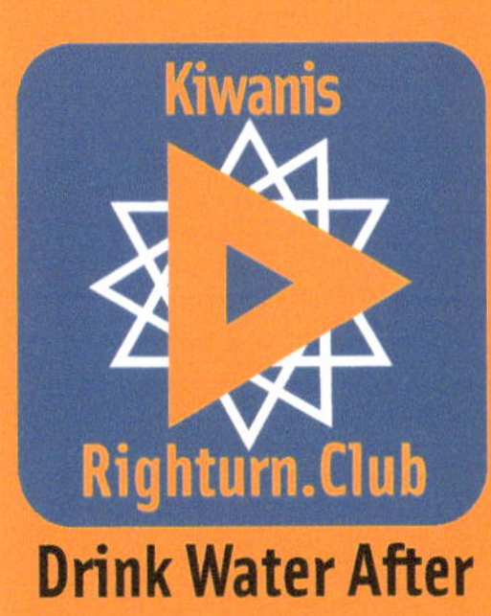

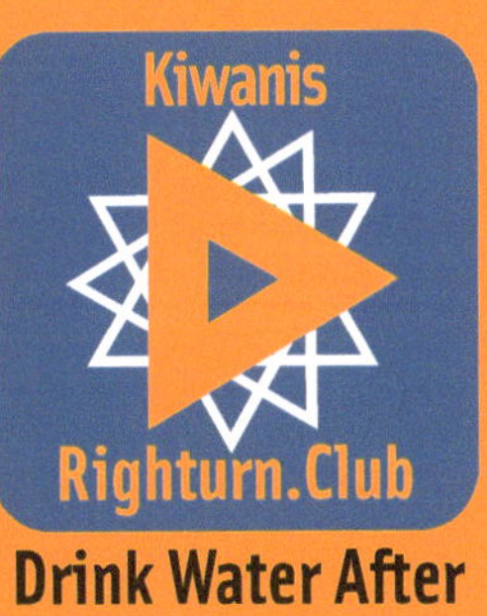

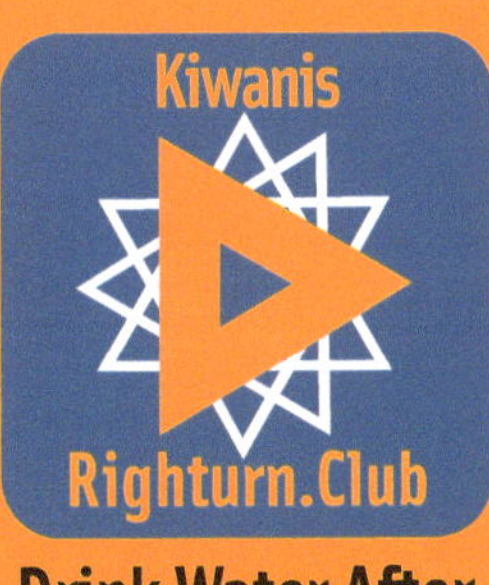

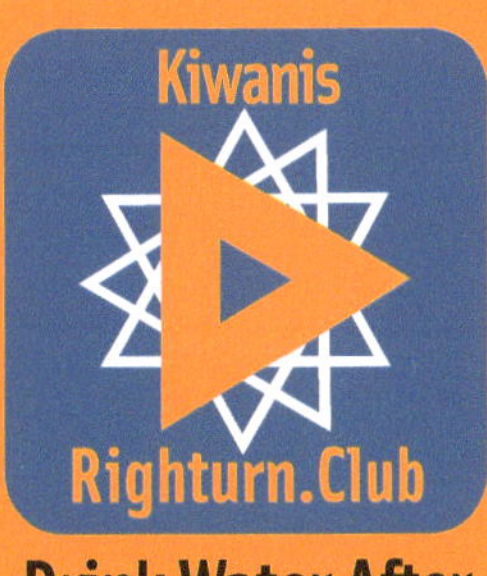

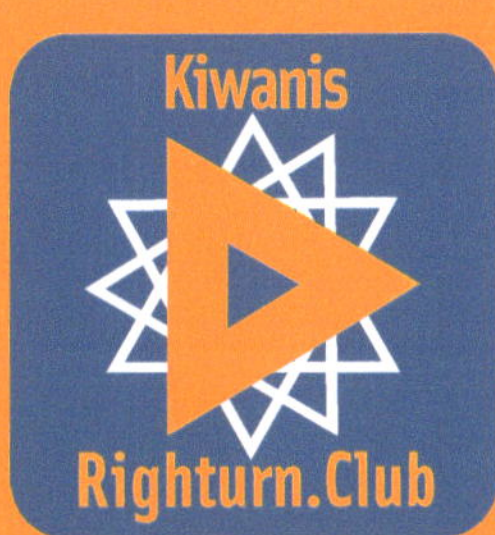

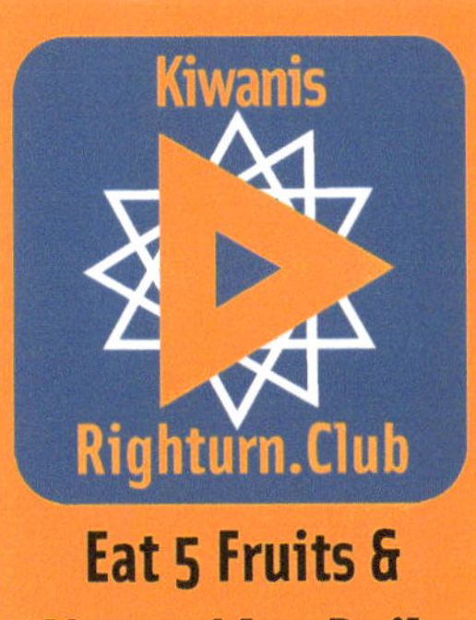

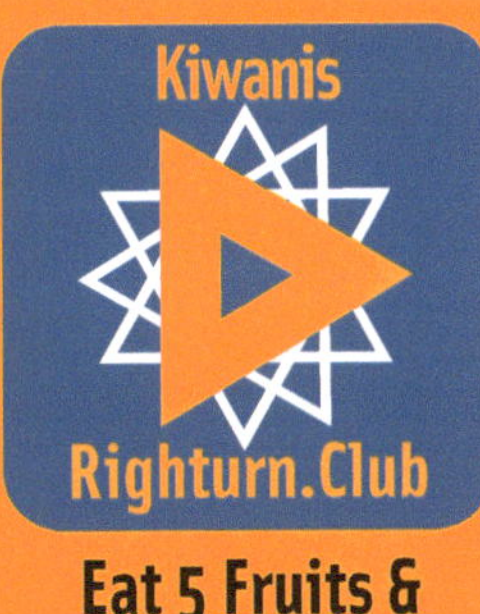

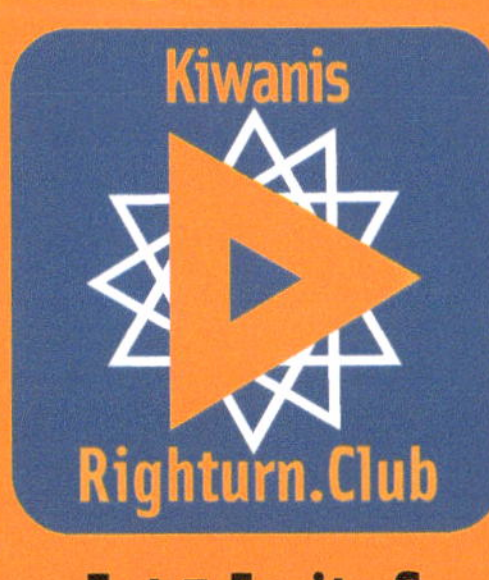

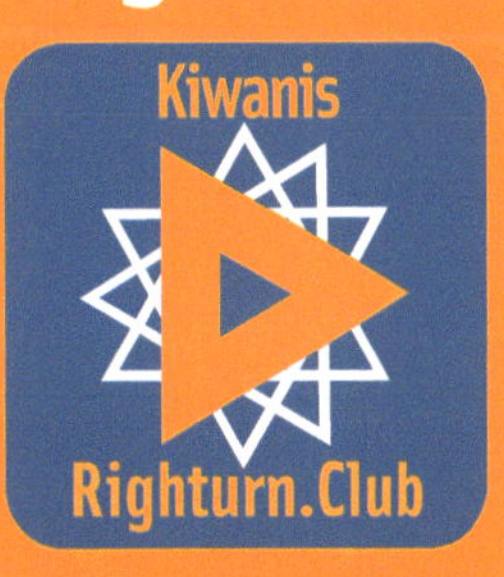

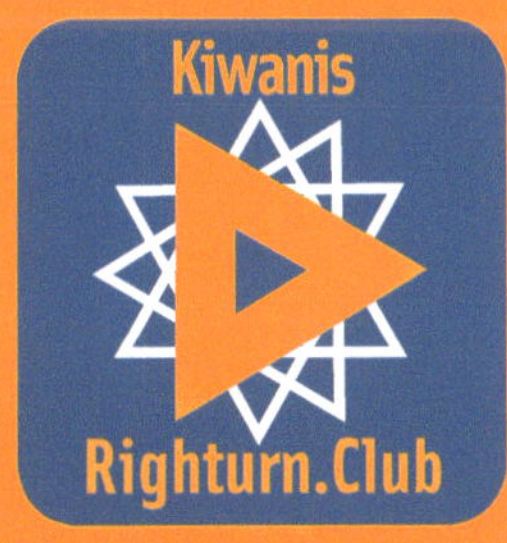

Giving Thanks

To _______________________

For your support, dedication and compassion
shown to the Kiwanis Righturn.Club

From _______________________
____

Kiwanis Righturn.Club

Giving Thanks

To _______________________

For your support, dedication and compassion
shown to the Kiwanis Righturn.Club

From _______________________
____

Kiwanis Righturn.Club

Thank You Cards: Print two up on a letter size cover stock paper, then trimmed: 8.5 x11in.

CHAPTER 9:
Special Recipies

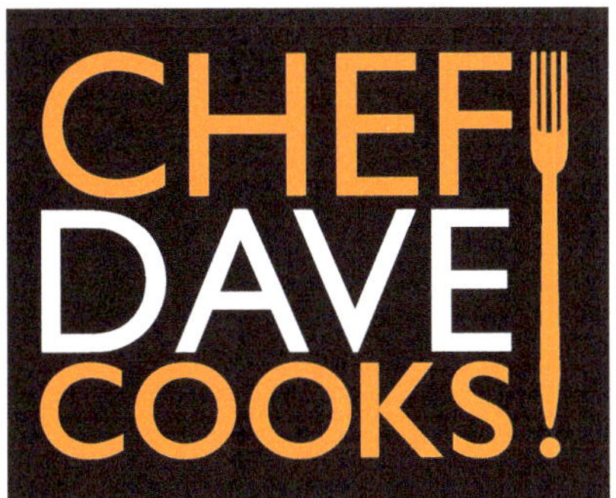

The following recipies are from Chef David Ingram, and include healthy ingredients. These can be used as a special treat for Righturn.Club kids. If you would like to share your special recipies from your club with other Righturn.Club kids, please send to Thomas@Moraitis.org.

▶ Mango Agua Fresca

5 1/2 cups Water
2 cups Mango Nectar, 100% juice, like Mango Tango
1/4 cup Agave Nectar
1/2 bunch Fresh Basil
Juice of 1 Lime

Place mango nectar, agave nectar, and basil in a blender and process about one minute. Pour through a fine mesh strainer into a pitcher or bowl and whisk basil pulp to get all the liquid through. Add water and lime juice and chill.

▶ Veggie Sandwich

2 slices Multi-grain Bread
1/2 Avocado (very ripe)
2 Tablespoons Almond, Cashew, or Peanut Butter
1 Roma Tomato, sliced thin
1/2 cup Alfalfa or other Sprouts
Red or green leaf lettuce
1 slice Provolone Cheese (optional)

Spread avocado on one slice of bread and sprinkle with a little salt and pepper if desired. Spread nut butter on other slice and layer rest of ingredients.

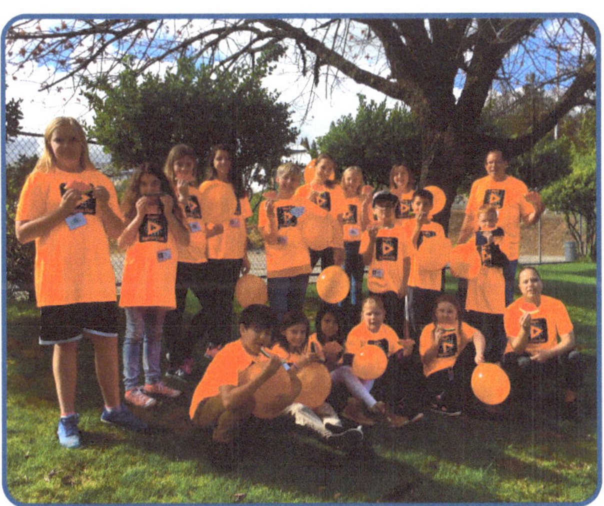

Kiwanis Righturn.Club kids having fun at Sutter Creek Elementary School, Spring 2017, Sutter Creek, CA.

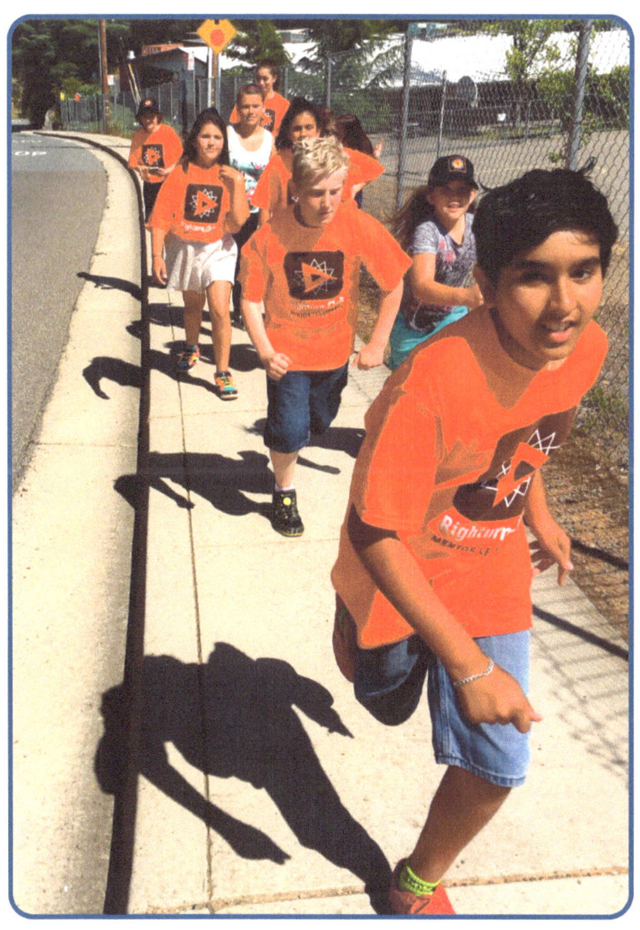

▶ Shrimp Cocktail

Sauce: 1 6oz.can Tomato paste

1/3 cup Apple Cider Vinegar

1 Tablespoon Worcestershire Sauce

1/2 cup Yellow Onion, chopped

2 ea. Garlic cloves

2 Tablespoons Prepared horseradish

1/4 cup Frozen Apple Juice Concentrate

Hot sauce or black pepper to taste

Place all ingredients in a blender and process until smooth. Chill.

For 4 cocktails: 6 cups Water

1 Tablespoon Seasoned Salt

16 ea. Easy-peel raw frozen Shrimp, 16/20 size

2 ribs Celery, diced

4 sprigs Parsley, chopped fine

4 ea. Lemon Wedges

1 1/3 cups Cocktail Sauce

Place water and salt in a 2 quart sauce pan and bring to a boil. Add shrimp and bring back to a boil then simmer for 1 minute. Drain, cool, and peel shrimp, then chill.

Mix celery and parsley together and divide between 4 bowls. Top with 1/3 cup of cocktail sauce, then shrimp and garnish with lemon wedges.

▶ Chocolate Mousse

Serves 4 to 6

16 oz. Tofu, extra firm (silken)

1/3 cup Evaporated milk (fat-free)

1/4 cup Agave Nectar

1/3 cup Dutch Process Cocoa Powder

2 teaspoons Vanilla Extract

Blend tofu and evaporated milk in a food processor until smooth. Add the rest of the ingredients and continue to process until creamy. You may need to scrape down the sides of the bowl a couple times. Pour into serving dishes and chill at least 4 hours

"Righturn.Club Rocks."
Thomas Moraitis

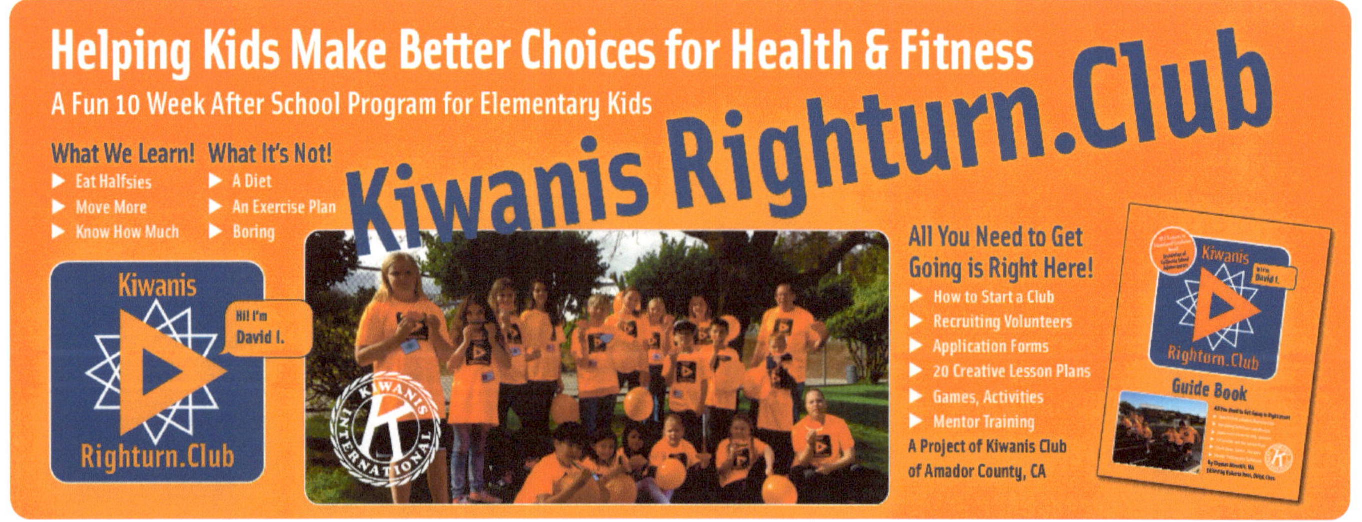

Banner:Size 48 in. Wide 18 in High

www.ingramcontent.com/pod-product-compliance
Lightning Source LLC
Chambersburg PA
CBHW040134240726
48664CB00002B/472